Clinical
Nephrology

2nd Edition

Woo Keng Thye

MBBS, M Med, FRACP, AM
Senior Consultant, Department of Renal Medicine
Singapore General Hospital;
Clinical Professor, National University of Singapore

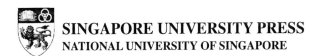
SINGAPORE UNIVERSITY PRESS
NATIONAL UNIVERSITY OF SINGAPORE

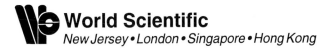
World Scientific
New Jersey • London • Singapore • Hong Kong

Published by

Singapore University Press
Yusof Ishak House, National University of Singapore
31 Lower Kent Ridge Road, Singapore 119078

and

World Scientific Publishing Co. Pte. Ltd.
P O Box 128, Farrer Road, Singapore 912805
USA office: Suite 1B, 1060 Main Street, River Edge, NJ 07661
UK office: 57 Shelton Street, Covent Garden, London WC2H 9HE

Library of Congress Cataloging-in-Publication Data
Woo, K. T. (Keng Thye)
    Clinical nephrology / Woo Keng Thye. -- 2nd ed.
        p. ; cm.
    Includes bibliographical references and index.
    ISBN 981238085X (pbk.)
    1. Kidneys -- Diseases.   2. Nephrology.   I. Title.
    [DNLM: 1. Kidney Diseases -- diagnosis -- Handbooks.   2. Kidney
    Diseases -- therapy -- Handbooks.   WJ 39 W873c 2002]
    RC902.W66 2002
    616.6'1--dc21   2002028845

British Library Cataloguing-in-Publication Data
A catalogue record for this book is available from the British Library.

Printed in Singapore by Uto-Print

For
May, Bernardine, Geraldine,
Bernard, Adeline and Anne.

My Teachers and Students,
past, present and future.

Yesterday this time, we sat at length
Analysed, dissected, polished ink stones
Bared the sinews of our thoughts
Between the bristles of the brush
And grains of rice-paper.

Preface

Over the past 30 years, Dr Woo has been teaching Renal Medicine to medical students and doctors. This book is written in response to their request to put together a series of tutorials and lectures in Renal Medicine to serve their needs for a textbook of Clinical Nephrology.

He has given a comprehensive review of Renal Medicine pertaining to Clinical Nephrology. The topics range from glomerulonephritis, urinary tract infection, hypertension and renal stones to renal failure, dialysis and transplantation, thus providing the student with a broad perspective of Renal Medicine. In addition, tables on local incidence and statistics are provided. This is important as all the available books on Renal Diseases have been written by overseas authors in the West, quoting data and statistics which are quite different from our local scene. Local data on disease incidence and patterns are important as there exist widely differing patterns of geographical distribution among various types of renal diseases in different parts of the world.

This book is also written for the practising doctor or clinician who is looking for a basic handbook to serve as a reference for current concepts and practice in clinical nephrology. It is written in simple language with discussions on clinical problems occurring in daily practice.

The knowledge in this book is graded. Many chapters will be relevant to medical students. However, depending on the requirements of the reader, whether he is a medical student or postgraduate doctor preparing for his M Med (Internal Medicine) Examination, he will be able to find within this book chapters relevant to his needs.

1st April 2002

Acknowledgements

It gives me great pleasure to acknowledge the contributions of the following:

Medical students and doctors whose needs have led me to write this book.

Ms Irene Ow for her secretarial assistance.

Mr Steven Patt, Editor, World Scientific Publishing, for his editorial assistance.

Clinical Associate Professor Gilbert Chiang, Senior Pathologist and Head, Singapore General Hospital, for his contribution in renal histopathology.

Contents

CHAPTER 1

Structure and Function

ANATOMY OF THE KIDNEYS

The kidneys are a pair of bean-shaped organs located at the back of the body about the level of the waist. They receive their blood supply from the main artery of the body called the aorta. Each kidney measures 10–15 cm in length and weighs about 160 gm. Urine is conducted from the kidneys along two tubes known as the ureters which join the urinary bladder in the pelvis. The capacity of the bladder varies from 500 to 750 ml. Each kidney is made up of 1 million units called nephrons. Each nephron consists of two parts, the glomerulus which is a bunch of capillaries with thin walls serving as a filter, and the tubule which drains the glomerulus (Figs. 1.1 & 1.2).

The glomerular tuft is made up of a coil of capillaries which is fed by an afferent arteriole and drained by an efferent arteriole. The tuft lies in a space known as Bowman's capsule which is spherical and opens directly into the proximal tubule. The glomerular tuft and capsule is lined by epithelial cells. Ultrafiltration occurs across the capillary tuft and the fluid passes into the proximal tubule. Between the afferent and the efferent arterioles of the glomerulus lies the juxta-glomerular apparatus which lies in the area bounded by the two arterioles, the distal tubule of the same nephron and the lacis cells lying between the two arterioles.

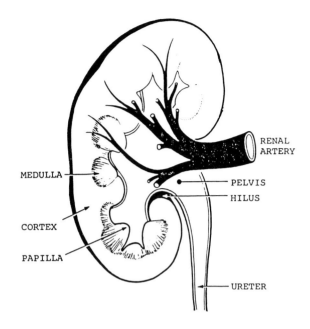

Fig. 1.1   The gross structure of the cut surface of the kidney

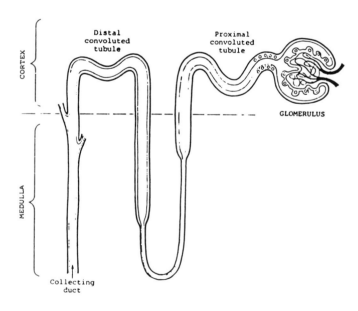

Fig. 1.2   Diagram of a nephron

Within the glomerular tuft are the mesangial cells and mesangial matrix. The mesangial cells have a supportive and phagocytic function and have been referred to as the third reticulo-endothelial system. They are capable of contraction and are involved in the pathogenesis of IgA nephritis and diabetic nephropathy. Factors or agents that cause increased mesangial cell contractility predispose to mesangial sclerosis and therefore glomerulosclerosis. The capillary loops abound around the core of mesangial cells and matrix. The wall of these capillary loops consists of three layers, the epithelial cells, the glomerular basement membrane and the endothelial cells (Fig. 1.3).

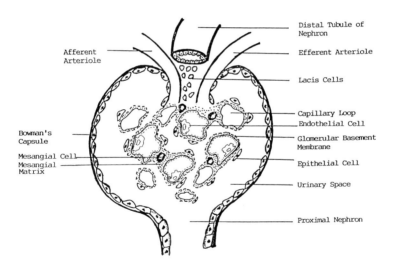

Fig. 1.3 Diagram of a glomerulus

The term "proliferative glomerulonephritis" refers to a proliferation of one of the three types of cells within the glomerulus: mesangial cells, endothelial cells or epithelial cells; and hence the different types of proliferative glomerulonephritis (GN): Mesangial Proliferative GN,

Endocapillary Proliferative GN and Crescenteric GN. In Crescenteric GN, there is now evidence to show that macrophages from the circulation as well as those in situ within the glomeruli gain entry into the glomerular tuft and transform themselves into epithelial cells and it is the proliferation of these transformed epithelial cells which forms the crescents in Crescenteric GN.

The glomerular basement membrane (GBM) is composed of three layers (notice that many things occur in "threes"): a central dense zone, known as the lamina densa, an inner and outer lucent zone, known respectively as the lamina rara interna and externa. The GBM is 80 nm thick.

Ultrastructural studies reveal that the "filtration barrier" is composed of an inner fenestrated endothelium, the GBM as the middle layer and the outer layer of interdigital epithelial foot processes.

Pores have never been visualised on the GBM which is biochemically a hydrated gel composed of collagen-like and non-collagenous glycoproteins. The non-collagenase glycoprotein is rich in hydroxyproline, galactose, mannose and sialic acid. The epithelial foot processes are covered by glycoproteins which are rich in sialic acid. The negative (anionic) charges of sialic acid help to keep the foot processes apart. The negative charges on the basement membrane (due to the presence of glycosaminoglycans, such as heparan sulphate) and around the epithelial slits (due to sialic acid), constitute a filtration barrier. This explains why the fractional clearance of negatively charged particles is less than that of neutral particles of similar molecular dimensions as negatively charged particles are repelled at the GBM. Positive (cationic) charges are attracted to the GBM. They interfere with the integrity of glomerular permselectivity (maintained by the negative charges) and induce proteinuria. Hence, positively charged particles have a higher fractional clearance than negatively charged particles.

Antibodies to the non-collagenous glycoproteins (which carry negative charges), but not antibodies to the collagenous glycoproteins, are nephrotoxic in experimentally induced anti-GBM nephritis.

Therefore it is not only the molecular size but also the electrostatic charge which determines a particle's exclusion from glomerular filtration. Loss of the charge barrier results in the loss of glomerular permselectivity and causes proteinuria.

FUNCTIONS OF THE KIDNEYS

Each day the two kidneys excrete about 1.5 to 2.5 litres of urine. One of the most important functions of the kidney is to regulate the amount of water and salt excreted. About 99% of the filtered salt is reabsorbed by the tubules. The output of salt is regulated to maintain a normal and constant salt level in the body. The renal tubules also reabsorb dissolved substances like glucose and amino acids, the building blocks of proteins. The kidney has the important task of ridding the body of excess acid and potassium.

There is a minimum amount of soluble waste we must excrete through our kidneys each day. They are mainly nitrogenous waste products, principally urea. These products are poisonous and they are the substances retained in the body when the kidney fails.

The kidney is also a producer of certain hormones. Renin is one of them. Renin by itself is inactive but it acts on angiotensin I to produce angiotensin II which causes blood vessels to constrict thereby raising the blood pressure. Another hormone produced by the kidney is the active form of vitamin D which is necessary for strong and healthy bones as it promotes the absorption of calcium from the bowels. Without it we suffer from rickets. Erythropoietin, the third hormone produced by the kidney is necessary for the formation of red blood cells in the bone marrow. Patients with diseased kidneys are anaemic because they lack erythropoietin. Prostaglandins, another hormone, regulates the blood flow and blood pressure.

The main function of the kidneys is to make urine which contains the waste products of our metabolic processes. By regulating the rate at which these substances are excreted the kidneys are able to maintain the internal environment or the "milieu interieur". The production of urine depends on the renal plasma flow and the glomerular filtration. Hence the measurement of the glomerular filtration rate (GFR) is an index of renal function.

In addition to various substances which are cleared by the kidneys, there are others which are filtered and reabsorbed like glucose and sodium, and some which are secreted or excreted by the renal tubules.

Renal Handling of Sodium

Sodium is filtered at the glomeruli and actively reabsorbed by the tubules. About 80% of filtered sodium chloride and water are reabsorbed by the proximal tubules. The sodium which reaches the distal tubule is reabsorbed by an ion exchange mechanism. Potassium and hydrogen ions are passed into the tubular lumen and sodium ions are removed actively from the lumen. This exchange mechanism is enhanced by aldosterone. Therefore, altogether about 99% of filtered sodium is reabsorbed. The volume of the extracellular fluid is determined by the sodium content of the body which is regulated by the kidneys.

Renal Handling of Potassium

The majority of potassium is reabsorbed in the proximal tubules and that which is found in the urine is derived from potassium exchanged for sodium which is reabsorbed in the distal tubules and the collecting ducts.

Kidney Regulation of Acid-Base Balance

Extracellular fluid is maintained at a pH between 7.35 to 7.45. Two forms of acid which are continuously produced by the body require buffering and subsequent excretion.

i. Carbon dioxide which is formed as a result of cellular metabolism combines with water to form carbonic acid. In the lungs, carbonic acid dissociates and CO_2 is eliminated in the expired air.

ii. Fixed acids are acids which cannot be excreted via the lungs. They are also produced by the body's metabolic processes. The hydrogen ions produced by these fixed acids are buffered by bicarbonate ions in the body. The role of kidneys is to "regenerate" the bicarbonate which has been used up in the buffering of fixed acids.

Acidification of the Urine and Excretion of H^+

In normal persons, renal acidification maintains the plasma bicarbonate at physiologic concentrations by reclaiming all the filtered bicarbonate and excreting endogenously produced non-volatile or fixed acids.

This mechanism takes place at 3 sites.

i. *At the Proximal Tubules:*

85% to 90% of filtered bicarbonate is reclaimed. For each mole of Na^+ reabsorbed, one mole of H^+ is excreted and one mole of bicarbonate is generated and returned to the blood.

Secreted H^+ titrates HCO^{3-} to H_2CO_3 in the tubular lumen.

$$H_2CO_3 \xrightarrow[\text{carbonic anhydrase}]{} H_2O + CO_2$$

ii. *At the Distal Tubule:*

10% to 15% of filtered bicarbonate is titrated with secreted H^+. The urine pH is now about 6.2. Also titrated are the urinary buffers:

$$Na_2HPO_4 \longrightarrow NaH_2PO_4$$
$$NH_3 \longrightarrow NH_4$$

Titratable Acid = Measure of H^+ excreted as NaH_2PO_4

iii. *At the Collecting Duct:*

5% of bicarbonate is reabsorbed. The secretory capacity for H^+ is small but the large gradient generated for H^+ secretion enables the kidney to reduce the urinary pH to values of 5 or less and excrete NH_4 and titratable acid at a rate equal to the endogenous production of the fixed acids.

Therefore

Net Acid Excretion = Titratable Acid + NH_4 – Bicarbonate excreted

In Metabolic Acidosis:

Bicarbonate is titrated to extinction in the proximal tubule. The secretion of H^+ at the distal tubule is not buffered by delivered bicarbonate as the gradient of H^+ at the lumen-peritubule is decreased. Urine pH is less than 5, net H^+ excretion is increased, but total H^+ secretion is decreased.

In Metabolic Alkalosis:

The amount of bicarbonate delivered to the distal tubule exceeds the H^+ secretory capacity. Urine pH is 8. Bicarbonaturia swamps H^+ excretion, though the total H^+ secretion is increased.

Adequacy of Gradient-Generating and Acid-Excreting Ability

The adequacy of gradient-generating and acid-excreting ability is evaluated by measurements of urinary pH, titratable acid and ammonium during metabolic acidosis, either spontaneous or induced by means of the ammonium chloride loading test (short or long test).

With small reduction in plasma bicarbonate concentration, eg. 3 to 4 mEq/l, normal subjects decrease urinary pH to less than 5.3, titratable acid increased to more than 25 and ammonium to more than 39 mEq per minute. Urine pH of 5.3 and below denotes ability to acidify the urine and urine pH above 5.3 denotes inability to acidify the urine.

In non-azotemic renal acidification defect, the urinary pH is high during acidosis and excretion rates of titratable acid and ammonium is reduced. The serum chloride increases as bicarbonate decreases. This defect is termed "Renal Tubular Acidosis" by Pines and Mudge.

Concentration of Urine

There is a progressive increase in tissue osmolarity from cortex to papillary tip. In the kidney the loops of Henle function as countercurrent multipliers. Fluid in the descending limb becomes progressively more concentrated during its passage from the cortico-medullary junction to the tip of the loop. In the ascending limb, sodium is reabsorbed more rapidly than water and the fluid passing to the distal convoluted tubule is more dilute than that which enters the descending limb. A gradient between the limbs is created by the transport of sodium unaccompanied by equivalent amounts of water out of the ascending limb into the interstitial fluid. Water then diffuses out of the descending limb so concentrating the contents of the limb until an equilibrium is reached in which the concentration of the fluid at any point in the descending limb is the same as that of the interstitial fluid at the same level and slightly higher than that at the corresponding point of the ascending limb.

The collecting ducts pass through the medulla. In the presence of antidiuretic hormone (ADH), water diffuses from the collecting ducts into the hypertonic medullary interstitium. This makes the urine progressively concentrated.

Also under the influence of ADH the collecting ducts, normally not permeable to urea, become highly permeable to urea. Urea diffuses from the collecting ducts into the medullary interstitial fluid. The urea trapped in the medullary interstitium extracts water from the descending limb of the loop of Henle and amplifies the effect of the counter-current multiplier. This permits the production of a more highly concentrated urine.

Hormones and the Kidneys

Many hormones influence various aspects of renal function. These are antidiuretic hormone, cortisol, aldosterone, parathyroid hormone, growth hormone, sex hormones, erythropoietin, prostaglandins and angiotensin II.

The autoregulation of renal blood flow maintains and regulates the GFR. Changes in the mean arterial pressure can induce changes in the opposite directions of afferent and efferent arteriolar resistances, resulting in near constancy of the GFR. For example, a reduction in systemic arterial pressure produces dilatation of afferent arterioles thus increasing the blood flow to the glomeruli and maintaining the perfusion pressure. However, if the efferent arterioles also dilate, the pressure will be transmitted to the post-glomerular capillary bed and GFR will decrease.

Vasoconstriction of the efferent arteriole is achieved by intrarenal generation of angiotensin II. The juxta-glomerular apparatus senses the perfusion pressure by means of stretch receptors in the afferent arteriole. A decrease in systemic arterial pressure releases renin from afferent arterioles.

In glomerular hyperfiltration, there is afferent arteriolar dilatation with increase of blood flow to the glomerulus. At the efferent arteriole, angiotensin II receptors induce vasoconstriction. The end result is increase in intraglomerular blood pressure (intraglomerular hypertension). This causes increase in single nephron GFR with increase in creatinine clearance and proteinuria. With time, however, the intraglomerular hypertension induces glomerulosclerosis. Hyperfiltration occurs in any condition where some glomeruli are sclerosed. Hyperfiltration or hyperperfusion then occurs in the remnant glomeruli. This condition occurs in diabetic nephropathy and IgA nephritis.

Prostaglandins play an essential role in normal renal function, especially PGE_2. Prostaglandins are located in the renal medulla. They modify the adenylcyclase cyclic AMP system and also have a role in regulation of renal blood flow and of ADH secretion and actions. Prostaglandins have also been implicated in hypertension. This is based on observations that a reduction in the renal production of certain types of prostaglandins is associated with reduced natriuresis and hypertension in experimental animals.

Other hormones like antidiuretic hormone (vasopressin) regulates water excretion. Cortisol promotes sodium retention and potassium and hydrogen loss by the kidneys. Aldosterone enhances the reabsorption of sodium from the distal tubular fluid in exchange for potassium and hydrogen ions which have increased excretion.

Parathyroid hormone diminishes the urinary output of calcium and hydrogen ions and increases that of phosphate and potassium ions. Growth hormone has some sodium retaining properties. Oestrogens may lead to salt and water retention and to a rise in GFR and renal blood flow in pregnancy. Progesterone induces sodium and water loss.

CHAPTER 2

Symptoms and Signs in Renal Medicine

HISTORY TAKING

1. **Pain:** Backache as a symptom of renal disease can be in the loin or over the lumbar spine. In renal colic due to renal stones the pain may start in the loin and radiate towards the groin and from there to the penis, sometimes even to the tip of the penis as in the case of a stone at the trigone of the urinary bladder. Suprapubic pain can be due to infection of the bladder (cystitis) or it could be due to a bladder stone. When pain is associated with fever or chills it is due to infection of the urinary tract.

2. **Swelling** due to oedema usually involves the extremities, ie. the face, the ankles and legs. There can be associated swelling of the abdomen (ascites) as in the case of the nephrotic syndrome. When swelling becomes generalised there is collection of fluid in the abdominal, pleural and even the pericardial space. This is referred to as anarsarca.

3. **Haematuria** or the presence of blood in the urine is said to be gross when it is apparent to the naked eye. It is microscopic when there are more than 3 red blood cells per high power field on urine microscopy. Enquire into the relationship of haematuria to renal stones or nephritis as in the acute nephritic syndrome which usually is associated with what is described as smoky urine in the case of post infectious glomerulonephritis. Post infectious

glomerulonephritis is also associated with a history of preceding sore throat. If gross haematuria occurs with sorethroat at the same time it is referred to as synpharyngitic haematuria and in the Singapore context this is a useful clue to the diagnosis of IgA nephritis, the commonest form of nephritis seen here. Haematuria in IgA nephritis may also be precipitated by exercise. Another cause of exercise induced haematuria is stress haematuria. This has now been found to be due to trauma to the blood vessels at the base of the bladder brought on by exercise or jogging.

4. **Dysuria** or pain on passing urine is due to infection of the bladder or the urethra (urethritis). Tuberculous cystitis or a tumour in the bladder can also give rise to dysuria.

5. **Strangury** is also painful micturition but in this case only a few drops of urine are passed. This is due to a severe inflammation of the bladder.

6. **Double micturition** is when a patient, soon after emptying the bladder wants to do so again. This occurs in patients with vesicoureteric reflux as they have a large residual urine volume in the bladder.

7. **Frequency of micturition** is when the patient passes urine many times over his normal micturition habits. This is often due to urinary tract infection.

8. **Nocturia** is when the patient awakes to pass urine a few times at night when previously he may usually do so only once at night. This is due either to urinary infection or it could be an early sign of renal failure as renal concentration is one of the earliest functions to be impaired in renal failure.

9. **Oliguria** refers to a decrease in urine output when the patient passes less than 400 ml of urine. This is a sign of renal failure.

10. **Anuria** is when there is absolutely no urine output. In this case acute renal failure due to an obstruction in the urinary tract has to be excluded. If obstruction is excluded, consider bilateral renal infarction due to thrombosis of the renal arteries or a descending dissecting aneurysm involving the renal arteries.

11. **Renal Failure:** The patient may complain of tiredness, shortness of breath, itch which is often generalised, poor appetite or anorexia, nausea, vomiting, giddiness, headache and swelling of the face and legs and passing scanty urine.

12. **Woman:** In the case of a female patient, enquire about her previous pregnancies, whether there was a history of swelling during pregnancy, protein in the urine and hypertension as this may suggest toxaemia of pregnancy. In the case of a woman with symptoms of urinary infection, enquire about the relationship to sexual activity.

13. **Man:** In a male patient with urinary infection, enquire about exposure to venereal disease and think of prostatic infection.

14. **System Review:** Ask for history of rashes, alopecia or joint pains as these may be clues to systemic lupus erythematosus. Does the patient have a cough or history of tuberculosis? This may be useful when suspecting renal tuberculosis. Fever together with weight loss may mean a cancer. Renal cell carcinoma is one of the causes of pyrexia of unknown origin. If the patient is an elderly lady with urinary infection and renal failure, one should perform a vaginal examination to exclude cancer of the cervix.

15. **Past and Family History** of kidney disease, childhood nephritis and urinary infection. If the patient had a history of kidney disease what investigations were performed?

Enquire about treatment and follow-up. Was there a family history of hypertension or diabetes mellitus?

16. Finally: Does the patient take **drugs** like analgesics (non-steroidal anti-inflammatory drug or NSAID) or traditional *sin-seh's* (Chinese physician) medicine which may do harm to the kidneys? Was there a history of recent instrumentation like in the case of those with catheter fever? Occupational hazards: A sewage or farm worker may contract leptospirosis; lead or hydrocarbon exposure may cause nephritis.

PHYSICAL EXAMINATION OF THE RENAL MASS

The renal mass is felt in the loin and has a well-defined rounded lower border. It is felt bimanually and can be pushed from one hand to the other, ie. ballotable. The front hand should be pressed towards the hand at the loin immediately at the end of inspiration.

One may be able to get above it. This feature would exclude a splenic and hepatic mass.

The differential diagnosis of a renal mass are polycystic kidneys, hydronephrosis, amyloidosis and renal carcinoma.

As part of the examination one should auscultate for a renal bruit which is a clue to the presence of renal artery stenosis.

An Enlarged Kidney or a Spleen?

The spleen has a sharp edge as well as a splenic notch. The edge of a kidney is rounded and there is no notch.

The fingers can be passed between the upper end of the kidney swelling and the ribs. A renal mass is bimanually palpable.

There is a colonic resonance in front of the renal mass.

KIDNEY DISEASES IN SINGAPORE

1. **Glomerulonephritis** is one of the commonest causes of chronic renal failure. Chronic glomerulonephritis accounts for at least 29% of end stage renal disease.

2. **Diabetes mellitus:** causes diabetic nephropathy, urinary tract infection and hypertension. Diabetic nephropathy is the commonest cause of chronic renal failure in Singapore, accounting for 47% of end stage renal failure.

3. **Leptospirosis** is a common cause of acute renal failure. The patient may have fever, jaundice, conjunctival suffusion and calf tenderness.

4. **Systemic Lupus Erythematosus** affects mainly young women. It causes lupus nephritis and presents as acute nephritic syndrome, nephrotic syndrome or asymptomatic urinary abnormalities. It is a cause of acute as well as chronic renal failure.

5. **Henoch-Schonlein purpura** causes nephritis and is associated with a purpuric rash over the buttocks and lower limbs.

6. **Urinary tract infection:** acute and chronic pyelonephritis, cystitis, prostatitis, urethritis.

7. **Renal stones, hydronephrosis, medullary sponge kidneys, renal tubular acidosis**.

8. **Adult polycystic kidneys:** usually bilateral; causes chronic renal failure in the older age group.

9. **Gout:** causes joint pains, renal stones, urinary infection and hypertension.

10. **Hypertension:** renal and essential hypertension are common. Kidney failure results from malignant and accelerated hypertension.

11. **Tuberculosis** is a cause of sterile pyuria with tuberculous pyelonephritis. It also presents with haematuria.

12. **Prostatic diseases:** hypertrophy of the prostate is a cause of obstructive uropathy and urinary tract infection.

13. **Cancer:** hypernephroma or renal cell carcinoma can present as a renal mass, painless haematuria or fever of unknown origin.

14. **Pregnancy:** pre-eclampsia, pregnancy superimposed on preexisting glomerulonephritis, urinary tract infection are all complications that could result in deterioration of renal function with renal failure as the outcome.

15. **Drugs:** analgesics giving rise to analgesic kidney with renal failure; non-steroidal anti-inflammatory drugs (NSAID) like indomethacin, brufen, ponstan, rofecoxib (vioxx) etc. can all cause acute renal failure by inhibiting prostaglandin synthesis. Traditional *sin-seh's* medicine too is a cause of tubulotoxic acute renal failure.

URINE EXAMINATION

The following should be noted, viz. colour, reaction (pH), specific gravity, sugar, albumin, blood, deposit (urine microscopy) — RBC, WBC, other cells, casts.

Further Remarks on Haematuria

Haematuria or the passage of bloody urine is a danger signal that cannot be ignored. Enquire about associated dysuria, vesical symptoms and whether there is blood throughout the urinary stream.

Exclude red urine after beets, laxatives, colouring agent rhodomine B in which case the urine would be translucent rather than opaque because of the absence of red blood cells. Haemoglobinuria due to the haemolysis of red blood cells also gives rise to red urine.

Symptoms and Diagnosis

1. Haematuria with renal colic could be due to a stone, clot colic or renal tumour.

2. Terminal haematuria could be due to tuberculosis of the bladder, bladder stone or prostatic bleeding.

3. A tumour of the bladder ulcerates and presents with infection and bleeding, ie. cystitis with haematuria.

4. Prostatic hypertrophy may be associated with dilated veins at the bladder neck which ruptures when the patient strains.

5. Haematuria without other symptoms or "silent" haematuria could be due to a tumour of the bladder or kidney. Bleeding may be intermittent and stops for months before recurring.

6. Staghorn calculus, polycystic kidneys, renal cyst may also cause haematuria.

7. Stress haematuria is caused by exertion, usually after jogging or running for long distances. This is due to trauma of blood vessels at the base of the bladder.

8. Glomerulonephritis like IgA nephritis can also be associated with haematuria on exertion or haematuria can be precipitated by an upper respiratory infection, gastroenteritis or any fever. Urine phase contrast microscopy will show dysmorphic RBC in these cases. In contrast, bleeding due to a stone or vascular cause will show isomorphic RBC under the phase contrast microscope.

Time of Haematuria

Try to determine if haematuria occurs at the initial part of the micturition stream, terminally or throughout micturition in order to facilitate the localisation of the site of haematuria.

Haematuria occurring at the initial portion could be due to some cause at the anterior urethra (urethritis, urethral stricture or meatal stenosis). Terminal haematuria could be due to posterior urethritis or a lesion at the bladder neck or trigone (polyps or tumours). Haematuria present throughout micturition means that the lesion is above the urinary bladder and could be due to a stone, tumour, tuberculosis or nephritis.

CHAPTER 3

Renal Investigations

A proper evaluation of kidney functions consists of the following:

1. Urine examination
2. Quantitative measurement of proteinuria
3. Glomerular function
4. Tubular function

URINE EXAMINATION

Urinary Red Blood Cells (RBC)

Under bright field microscopy, normal urine contains not more than 3 red blood cells (RBC) or white blood cells (WBC) per high power field (hpf). Apart from hyaline casts, other types of casts like RBC casts, granular or broad waxy casts should be absent. However, exercise can increase the number of cells and casts excreted, even in normal individuals and occasionally, granular casts are also excreted.

In patients presenting with haematuria it is particularly important to determine whether the bleeding is from a glomerular or non-glomerular source. This is now possible using Phase Contrast Microscopy. In glomerular bleeding (due to glomerulonephritis) the urinary RBC have a dysmorphic pattern. There is a profusion of RBC of bizarre shapes and dissimilar sizes. Normal centrifuged urine contains up to

8000 dysmorphic RBC per ml of urine. Increased number of dysmorphic RBC suggests a diagnosis of glomerular disease. The presence of concomitant proteinuria is another clue which points to a diagnosis of glomerular disease.

In non-glomerular bleeding associated with urinary calculus, tumours and papillary necrosis, the RBC are isomorphic (of uniform size and shape). A count as low as 4000 per ml is indicative of non-glomerular bleeding, and an intravenous pyelogram (IVP) may be required to exclude a stone or a cystoscopy required to exclude a tumour in the bladder.

Sometimes in patients with IgA nephritis or lupus nephritis, the patient may have a mixed pattern, ie. both glomerular and non-glomerular RBC.

Leukocytes

The presence of WBC (pyuria) indicates infection or interstitial nephritis. Look for associated squamous epithelial cells in a female patient. The presence of epithelial cells with WBC indicates contamination by vaginal secretions and not a true urinary infection.

Casts

RBC casts imply the presence of glomerular disease and WBC casts indicate pyelonephritis. Normal urine contains hyaline casts (< 100/ml of urine). However, diuretic treatment can increase the number of hyaline casts in normal individuals (up to 20,000/ml of urine). Granular casts, oval fat bodies and broad waxy casts suggest an underlying renal lesion. In normal subjects, casts are composed of Tamm Horsfall protein but in diseased states, casts are found from different cellular elements. Triamterene, a diuretic, can induce the formation of large brown bizarre casts containing triamterene crystals which can be mistaken for granular casts. However, triamterene casts and crystals will polarise when examined under polarised light.

QUANTITATIVE MEASUREMENT OF PROTEINURIA

Absence of significant proteinuria is a sign of renal integrity and its presence indicates renal disease. In normal individuals the 24-hour urinary protein is less than 150 mg per day.

Proteinuria could be due to:

1. Increased glomerular filtration because of increased permeability of basement membrane.
2. Decreased reabsorption of proteins.
3. Addition of protein to urine (renal tubular cells, lymphatics, genitalia). In Bence Jones proteinuria, there are abnormal light chains which coagulate on heating at a temperature of 45° to 55°C and redissolve on boiling.

Protein selectivity refers to the ratio of the clearance of a large molecular weight protein like IgG to a smaller one like transferrin. Patients with nephrotic syndrome and selective proteinuria tend to respond to therapy with steroids as opposed to those with non-selective proteinuria. In our experience, patients with Minimal Change nephrotic syndrome and those with mild diffuse mesangial proliferative glomerulonephritis tend to respond to prednisolone or cyclophosphamide therapy when they have selective proteinuria.

Proteinuria is greater during the day than at night and increases during upright position and exercise.

A reduction of proteinuria may indicate an improvement of glomerular disease or it may mean increasing glomerulosclerosis allowing less protein to be filtered into the urine.

Intermittent proteinuria may signify developing or healing lesions.

Persisting proteinuria of more than 1 gm a day indicates a less benign glomerular lesion on renal biopsy.

Functional proteinuria can be due to exercise or fever, extreme heat or cold.

Postural proteinuria occurs in 3 to 5% of healthy individuals. It is mild during the upright position and disappears on recumbence. The upright posture with lordosis causes renal venous congestion with decreased renal blood flow and proteinuria.

GLOMERULAR FUNCTION

Clinical measurement of renal function for:

1. Detecting disease
2. Evaluating its severity
3. Following its progress
4. Safe and effective use of drugs excreted by the kidney

Blood Urea Level

Urea production is rapidly affected by protein intake. It fluctuates more widely than creatinine.

When protein catabolism is increased, urea rises rapidly as in haemorrhage in the bowels or body tissues, severe infections, burns, muscle injury, ingestion of steroids and tetracycline (except doxycycline). Urea level falls with a low protein diet, starvation and liver damage.

Factors Affecting Serum Creatinine

1. Increase
   — large muscle mass
   — diet rich in meat
   — ketones, drugs (cephalosporin, aldactone, aspirin, co-trimoxazole)

2. Decrease
   — reduced muscle mass
   — severe renal failure causes decreased muscle mass, increased tubular secretion and intestinal destruction of creatinine

3. Variable — due to laboratory error

Glomerular Filtration Rate (GFR)

Renal blood flow (RBF) and GFR are maintained over a wide range of renal arterial pressures by altering the tone in afferent and efferent arterioles. The GFR is maintained by net filtration pressure and permeability of membrane.

GFR is the most widely used test of renal function. Ideally, it is measured using a substance which is:

1. eliminated only by the kidney
2. freely filtered

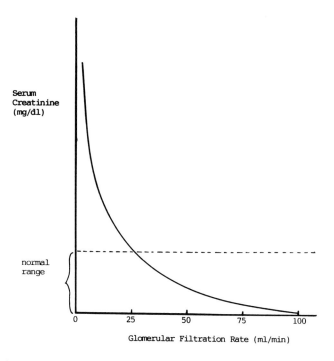

Fig. 3.1   Relationship between glomerular filtration rate and serum creatinine

3. neither secreted nor absorbed by tubules
4. easily and accurately measured

Fig. 3.1 shows the relationship between serum creatinine and GFR.

Measurement of GFR

Inulin Clearance

1. GFR as measured by inulin clearance is a research tool. Its accuracy is therefore a gold standard.

2. For the test, infuse inulin for 3 hours to ensure a steady concentration in the extracellular fluid (ECF).
3. Maintain a high fluid intake.
4. At equilibrium, the amount of inulin filtered by the glomerulus (GFR × P) equals the amount excreted in the urine (U × V).

$$GFR = \frac{U \times V}{P} = \frac{U \times Volume}{P \times T \ (Time)}$$

Creatinine Clearance

1. The endogenous production of creatinine by muscle metabolism is constant and proportional to the muscle mass.
2. There is a slight amount secreted by the tubules but common methods slightly overestimate plasma concentration.
3. A 24-hour urine collection is necessary. This urine specimen is also useful for quantitation of urinary protein.
4. The GFR varies inversely with the plasma concentration.

Chromium^{51}-EDTA

1. There is a small extra renal clearance which slightly underestimates the GFR.
2. Clearance is obtained using an intravenous infusion and timed urine collection, as for inulin.
3. A single intravenous injection is given which diffuses quickly into the ECF.
4. After the initial drop, plasma radioactivity falls exponentially. The slope is determined by the line of the GFR.
5. For calculation: slope of line multiplied by volume of distribution. The volume of distribution is determined by injected dose divided by plasma activity at zero time.

Estimation of GFR by Radiopharmaceuticals

1. Chromium[51] -EDTA
2. Iodine[125] sodium iothalamate
3. 99m technetium DTPA

These are gamma emitting isotopes. They are easily measured and there is no need for urine sample or collection.

Estimation of GFR Using Beta 2 Microglobulin

1. Beta 2 microglobulin is a surface constituent of most cells.
2. It is present in plasma in low concentration and is a low molecular weight protein of 11,800 daltons.
3. It is filtered freely at the glomerulus and is reabsorbed by cells of the proximal tubules.
4. B2m is produced at a constant rate and is not affected by muscle mass or diet.
5. It is measured by means of a radioimmunoassay.

TUBULAR FUNCTION

I. Proximal tubular function is assessed by reabsorption of glucose, phosphate, urate and amino acids.

II. Distal tubular function is assessed by urine concentration, dilution and acidification.

Proximal Tubular Function

1. Four functions are commonly assessed — reabsorption of glucose, phosphate, urate and amino acids.

2. Urine glucose, plasma phosphate, plasma urate and urinary amino acids are measured.

Amino Acids

a. Amino acids are freely filtered at the glomerulus and are almost completely reabsorbed by the proximal tubule.
b. The commonest are cystine, ornithine, lysine and arginine.
c. Proximal tubular lesions cause generalised or isolated amino acid leak.
d. Two-dimensional chromatography can be used to detect the leak.
e. In patients with cystinuria, the excretion of cystine is measured.

Urate

a. If plasma urate (serum uric acid) concentration is low, perform simultaneous measurement of 24-hour urate and creatinine clearance.
b. In the presence of low or normal plasma urate; a urate clearance:creatinine clearance ratio of over 10% indicates a tubular leak.

Phosphate

a. If plasma phosphate is consistently low or at the lower limit of the normal level, carry out simultaneous measurement of phosphate and creatinine clearance.
b. If the plasma phosphate is low and the phosphate clearance: creatinine clearance ratio is high (> 20%), this is evidence of proximal tubular dysfunction.

Glycosuria

a. This is tested for in random urine samples throughout the day.

b. Simultaneous measurement of plasma glucose is performed if any urine sample contains glucose.

c. Glycosuria without hyperglycaemia indicates proximal tubular malfunction.

Urinary Concentration Ability

1. Specific gravity
   If the morning urine has a SG of 1.018 or more, no further test is necessary as it implies normal concentration ability.

2. Osmolality
   If the early morning urine has an osmolality > 550 mOsmol/kg, no further test is necessary.

   If the osmolality is < 550 mOsmol/kg, further investigation is required.

Maximal Osmolar Concentration

1. After an overnight fast, give pitressin tannate 5 units subcutaneously or 20 μgm intranasally of desmopressin in each nostril.

2. Urine osmolality is measured hourly for 8 hours or until a sufficiently concentrated sample of urine is obtained before that.

3. An osmolality of 800 mOsmol/kg is accepted as normal.

Impaired Urinary Concentration

The following are possible causes:

1. high plasma calcium
2. low plasma potassium
3. protein malnutrition
4. prolonged high fluid intake
5. diabetes insipidus
6. drugs (eg. lithium)

Dilution Test

This is a measure of tubular functional integrity. Usually, the ability of the kidneys to concentrate urine is lost before its diluting ability. Complaints about nocturia is a signal that there may be a defect in concentration. At this stage the patient has polyuria and passes a dilute urine. Later on with further renal damage and with decreased renal perfusion, the patient passes less urine (oliguria).

1. For the test, the patient drinks 1 litre of fluid over 30 minutes. Urine is collected over 3 hours.
2. A normal person should excrete more than 50% of the volume in 3 hours.
3. The SG in one of the urine samples should be less than 1.003.

Urinary Acidification

1. No test is required if the overnight urine pH is 5.3 or less.
2. A plasma bicarbonate of less than or equal to 20 mEq/l is sufficient stimulus to acidify the urine.

3. Urine pH should be 5.3 or less in the Ammonium Chloride Loading Test.

Short Test of Wrong and Davis

1. Ammonium chloride, 100 mg/kg body weight is given in capsules or in a flavoured mixture at breakfast.
2. The pH is measured in all urine samples collected over 8 hours.
3. Blood samples are taken at the start and the end of the test to confirm a significant fall in plasma bicarbonate. This is to check that patient has not vomited the ammonium chloride ingested.
4. At least one urine sample should have pH 5.3 or less.
5. Titratable acid and ammonium excretion are also measured at the same time.
6. Refer to chapter on Renal Tubular Acidosis for more details.

RENAL FUNCTION WITH INCREASING AGE

1. There is a gradual decrease in all aspects of renal function after the age of 40 years.
2. This is due to involution and renal vascular degeneration.
3. There is a reduction in GFR which is accompanied by a decrease in muscle mass with age. Hence there is little change in the serum creatinine. Therefore if the GFR is not simultaneously measured with the serum creatinine, it may be presumed that the person still has his normal renal reserve (normal GFR).
4. In this instance if the person is given the normal dose of digoxin or an aminoglycoside antibiotic without being aware that in fact his GFR is lower than presumed (in the

presence of still normal serum creatinine), he will run the risk of drug toxicity as well as nephrotoxicity.

This explains why older patients with apparently normal serum creatinine who are given a dose of gentamicin 80 mg or 60 mg three times a day often develop renal impairment (as evidenced by a rise in serum creatinine) soon after. It is therefore useful to remember that old people with apparently normal serum creatinine in fact do not have "normal" renal function.

CHAPTER 4

Glomerulonephritis

The term glomerulonephritis refers to an inflammation of the kidneys.

The major clinical syndromes are:

1. Acute nephritic syndrome
2. Rapidly progressive glomerulonephritis
3. Persistent urinary abnormalities
4. Nephrotic syndrome
5. Nephritic nephrotic syndrome

Glomerulonephritis may be:

1. Primary or idiopathic
2. Secondary to multisystem diseases

Table 4.1 shows the histological distribution of Primary Glomerulonephritis (GN) occurring in Singapore. Comparing the data before and after 1990, diffuse mesangial proliferative GN (DPGN) is still the most common form of glomerulonephritis but it has decreased from 52% to 35% with an increase in all other forms of GN. This is the result of a change in the renal biopsy policy of the Department. Before 1990, patients with more than a gram of proteinuria were biopsied but after 1990, only those with more than 2 gm of proteinuria were biopsied apart from other criteria. This would mean that many patients with proteinuria of less than 2 gm were not biopsied and majority of them would be

Table 4.1 Primary Glomerulonephritis in Singapore

	(1976–1989)		(1990–1997)	
	No. of Cases	%	No. of Cases	%
1. Diffuse Mesangial Proliferative GN	768	52%	169	35%
2. Focal GN	131	9%	58	12%
3. Minimal Lesion	148	10%	70	14%
4. Focal Global Sclerosis	140	9%	65	13%
5. Focal & Segmental Sclerosis (FSGS)	119	8%	57	12%
6. Membranous GN	67	4%	30	6%
7. Others	112	8%	40	8%
TOTAL	1485	100%	489	100%

those with DPGN with IgA nephritis forming the predominant group. Our policy now is to revert to the criterion of more than a gram of proteinuria for biopsy. Other criteria are as listed under the Indications for Renal biopsy. As a whole then, we cannot state categorically that the profile of primary GN has not changed very much. Therefore the data before 1990 is more representative of the profile of primary GN in Singapore.

The other observation is that among the group with Focal Global Sclerosis; the indications for biopsy in many were Hypertension or Proteinuria. This group is believed to comprise a significant number of patients with Essential Hypertension who have Hypertensive Nephrosclerosis. (Refer to Chapter on Hypertension).

ACUTE NEPHRITIC SYNDROME

The features are oedema with gross haematuria (smoky urine) and frequent association with hypertension. Sometimes the symptoms are complicated by encephalopathy and congestive heart failure. This condition may be caused by bacteria, parasites, viruses, systemic lupus erythematosus, Henoch-Schonlein purpura and Guillain-Barre syndrome.

Post streptococcal glomerulonephritis which classically presents as the nephritic syndrome is better referred to as Post Infectious Glomerulonephritis because apart from streptococci, other bacteria and viruses can be the causative agent. It affects children principally, but no age is exempt. There is usually a latent period of 10 to 21 days. The urine characteristically shows a rusty or smoky hue. Mild renal impairment is common. Serum Complements (CH50 and C3) are usually low but normalises after 6 to 8 weeks.

Renal biopsy in patients with post infectious glomerulonephritis shows diffuse endocapillary proliferative glomerulonephritis with exudation of polymorphonuclears (acute exudative glomerulonephritis) (see Fig. 4.1). Electron microscopy (EM)

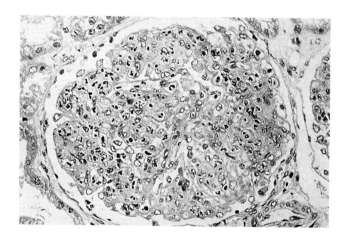

Fig. 4.1   Endocapillary glomerulonephritis. There is proliferation of endocapillary cells with polymorph infiltration. HE Stain original magnification 300X

shows subepithelial humps. Immunofluorescence (IMF) shows IgG often with C3. Sometimes IgA and IgM may be present in smaller amounts.

Treatment is usually symptomatic: generally bed rest is recommended during the acute phase. Restrict fluids and salt if oedema is present. Treat accompanying hypertension and heart failure. A course of Penicillin is given if throat swab grows streptococci. Dialysis may be required in some instances to tide the patient over the acute renal failure which may complicate the course of a few patients.

For the majority of patients, this is a benign disease, with children faring better than adults. Glassock[1] reported a 99% 5-year and a 97% 10-year survival for children whereas adults have 95% 5-year and a 90% 10-year survival. Potter[2] in a series of 534 patients from Trinidad followed up for 12 to 17 years reported only 2 deaths from chronic renal failure. Both those patients had persistent urinary abnormalities. Of the surviving patients, 3.6% had urinary abnormalities and another 3.6% had hypertension. All had normal serum creatinine.

In a paper from Israel, Drachman[3] showed that 80% of an original group of 155 children followed up for 11 to 12 years had normal urinary findings and blood pressure. Singhal[4] however showed in his study from India that 25 out of 144 of his patients died within 2 years and another 6 had renal impairment. In the next 8 years, 6 others developed renal impairment and 3 end stage renal failure (ESRF).

The bad prognostic features in this disease are persistent nephrotic syndrome, hypertension, renal impairment and crescents. These bad prognostic features however, as we shall see later, are true for most forms of glomerulonephritis.

RAPIDLY PROGRESSIVE GLOMERULONEPHRITIS (CRESCENTERIC GLOMERULONEPHRITIS) (Fig. 4.2)

This is a clinical syndrome of rapid and progressive decline in renal function, usually resulting in end stage renal failure in weeks to months, where there is extensive and exuberant proliferation of epithelial cells of Bowman's space.

In clinical practice, this condition is diagnosed when a patient has a rapid decline in glomerular filtration rate (acute renal failure), usually with oliguria, haematuria, hypertension in the presence of normal sized or enlarged kidneys. A renal biopsy will show extensive crescents of more than 70%.

Preceding flu-like illness is found in 50% of patients. Hypertension is often mild. Urine microscopy shows many

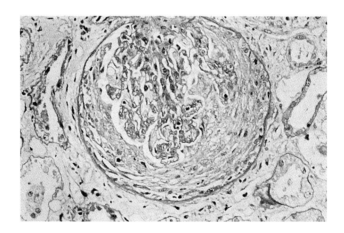

Fig. 4.2 Crescenteric glomerulonephritis. Crescent formation with compression of the glomerular tuft is seen. PAS Stain original magnification 300X

RBC with RBC casts. Serum complements (CH50, C3 and Clq) are often normal. Fibrin degradation products are often present and anti-streptolysin 0 titre is increased in 30% of patients.

Histology shows extensive extracapillary proliferation (crescents). IMF may show diffuse linear IgG, diffuse granular IgG, IgM and C3 or negative staining as in vasculitis. Fibrin related antigens are also present. Linear IgG with lung haemorrhage suggests Goodpasture's syndrome. Diffuse granular IgG indicates an immune complex glomerulonephritis like post streptococcal glomerulonephritis, systemic lupus erythematosus or nephritis due to subacute bacterial endocarditis.

Classify by absence or presence of glomerular Immune-Complexes (I.C)

(i)   Linear anti GBM antibody — Goodpasture's Syndrome
(ii) Granular Immune Complexes — SLE, HSP, SBE, PSGN
(iii) Pauci-immune Complexes — Wegener's Granulomatosis, Microscopic Polyarteritis Nodosa (PAN), Idiopathic Crescenteric GN

Treatment consists of plasmapheresis with steroids and cyclophosphamide, ideally administered prior to the onset of oliguria. A quadruple regimen with heparin, prednisolone, cyclophosphamide and anti-platelet agents (dipyridamole) has been used with success,[5] but caution should be exercised when using heparin. A low dose continuous heparin regimen during the acute phase to avoid haemorrhage, and then switch over to warfarin therapy is safer. A better alternative is to use pulse therapy with methyl prednisolone (0.5 gm I.V. daily for 6 days). Other measures include restriction of salt and water, treatment of hypertension and supportive dialysis.

This is a disease with a bad prognosis. The outlook for recovery is especially poor in the presence of:

1. circumferential crescents.
2. severe tubular atrophy and interstitial fibrosis.
3. extensive glomerular fibrosis and reorganisation of crescents, a late finding signifying irreversibility.
4. oliguria with a glomerular filtration rate of less than 5 ml per minute.

Patients with 50% to 80% crescents on biopsy have less than 30% 5-year and less than 10% 10-year survival. Those with 80% crescents have an 8% 5-year and less than 5% 10-year survival.

ASYMPTOMATIC HAEMATURIA AND PROTEINURIA

Asymptomatic haematuria and proteinuria is the most common presenting sign for a wide variety of glomerulonephritis. In the Singapore context, this is the usual presentation for IgA nephritis, the commonest form of glomerulonephritis occurring in Singapore. Patients with such urinary abnormalities are often referred by their general practitioners following a routine investigation for some unrelated complaints. Such cases are also detected on community health surveys or in the course of screening of national service registrants, for example, at the Central Manpower Base as in the case of Singapore. Surgeons too, often refer patients with asymptomatic haematuria after they have been shown to have normal intravenous pyelogram and cystoscopic examination.

History

One should ascertain that the patient is truly asymptomatic. Enquire for a history of gross or macroscopic haematuria, dysuria or frequency of micturition which may point to a diagnosis of haemorrhagic cystitis. A history of nocturia, backache, passage of stones, oedema or recurrent sore throat may provide useful clues to the underlying basis of urinary abnormalities.

If the patient has episodes of gross haematuria, determine if there is a relationship to upper respiratory tract infection, fever or exercise as IgA nephritis is associated with synpharyngitic haematuria, ie. gross haematuria occurring simultaneously with sore throat.

Always ask for a history of systemic illness. Tuberculosis, Systemic Lupus Erythematosus and Henoch-Schonlein purpura may present with urinary abnormalities. A family history of nephritis, hypertension and diabetes mellitus may be important. In a married woman, enquire into a past history of pre-eclampsia.

Physical Examination

In the general examination look for pallor, sallowness, presence of oedema and the rash of Henoch-Schonlein purpura or Systemic Lupus Erythematosus. Examine the abdomen for ballotable kidneys or renal masses which may suggest polycystic kidneys or a renal tumour. Always check the blood pressure, examine the fundi and listen for a renal bruit.

In most cases with asymptomatic haematuria and proteinuria the physical examination is usually normal; nevertheless a complete physical examination is mandatory to exclude any obvious underlying cause for the urinary abnormality.

Investigations

1. A full blood count and erythrocyte sedimentation rate (ESR) may be the first clues to SLE and tuberculosis.

2. Urine Microscopy
    i. RBC count is usually variable and may be anything from 5–10 to 100–300 per high power field.
    ii. WBC count: if pyuria is present, exclude urinary tract infection by doing a urine culture. For sterile pyuria, tuberculosis has to be excluded.
    iii. Casts: RBC casts point to a glomerulonephritis. Granular casts associated with more than a gram of proteinuria per day denotes a more severe lesion.
    iv. Albumin may vary from trace to 3 plus.

3. Quantitation of total urinary protein (TUP) in 24 hours. Normally this should not exceed 0.15 gm. In our experience, a TUP of more than 1 gm generally denotes a more severe glomerular lesion on renal biopsy, ie. the presence of glomerular scarring (glomerulosclerosis).

4. Blood urea, serum creatinine and creatinine clearance should be documented.

5. Lupus erythematosus (LE) cell and anti-nuclear factor (ANF) should be done when one suspects SLE together with Anti-DNA and Serum Complement.

Mild microscopic haematuria (< 20 RBC/high-power field (hpf)) in the absence of significant proteinuria is of little prognostic significance. In our experience, renal biopsies of this group of patients usually reveal only mild glomerulonephritis, which generally, has a good prognosis.

Sometimes on follow-up, patients may develop gross haematuria that may be precipitated by respiratory tract infections or exercises. Such patients on biopsy usually have IgA nephritis.

Proteinuria of 1 gm or more is an indication for a renal biopsy. Biopsy is performed under ultrasound guidance.

The intravenous pyelogram usually shows normal kidneys in patients with asymptomatic haematuria and proteinuria. If there is bilaterally symmetrical contracted kidneys it means that the patient probably has chronic glomerulonephritis. The presence of irregular scarring with calyceal distortion denotes chronic atrophic pyelonephritis due to vesico-ureteric reflux. Localised strictures of the calyces may be a clue to tuberculosis. The IVP may sometimes reveal polycystic kidneys, renal cysts or a renal tumour.

Indications for Renal Biopsy

Renal biopsy should be considered in patients with asymptomatic haematuria and proteinuria if they have:

1. Proteinuria of 1 gm or more.
2. Urine RBC persistently greater than 100 per hpf.
3. Gross haematuria on follow-up, associated with heavy proteinuria.
4. Presence of abnormal renal function or hypertension.

Renal Biopsy

Specimens are processed for light microscopy, immuno-fluorescence and electron microscopic studies.

1. Mesangial proliferative glomerulonephritis (focal or diffuse) with or without glomerulosclerosis is the commonest lesion in patients with asymptomatic haematuria and proteinuria. IMF studies show positive staining for IgA and EM studies

show mesangial electron dense deposits. In other words, such patients have Mesangial IgA nephritis. This is the commonest form of glomerulonephritis occurring here.

Tables 4.2 and 4.3 show the presenting features and histopathology of patients with IgA nephritis (see Fig. 4.3, 4.4 & 4.5). Table 4.2 shows that the group presenting with Asymptomatic Haematuria and Proteinuria has decreased comparing data before and after 1990. This again can be explained by the 2 gm of proteinuria criterion for renal biopsy as many with Asymptomatic Haematuria and Proteinuria with less than 2 gm would not be biopsied. In proportion therefore the other groups would be increased. At face value, the data from 1990 show an increase in those with nephrotic syndrome, acute nephritis and hypertension. The decrease in those with renal failure could mean that patients are coming earlier for medical screening and hence earlier detection. The decrease in those with gross haematuria subjected to renal biopsy may reflect our reluctance to biopsy this group of patients as they have a good prognosis in the absence of significant

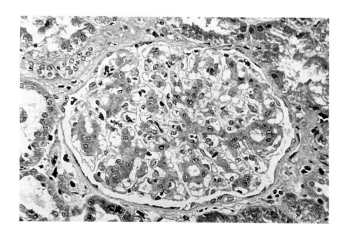

Fig. 4.3   IgA nephropathy. Increase in mesangial matrix and cells are seen. HE Stain original magnification 300X

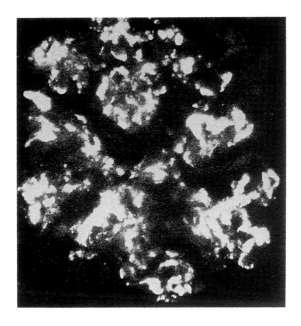

Fig. 4.4 IgA nephropathy. Deposits of IgA are seen on immunofluorescence. Original magnification 300X

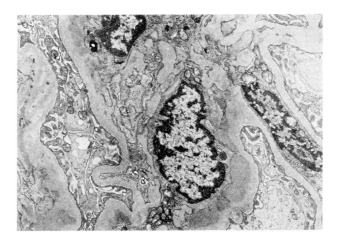

Fig. 4.5 IgA nephropathy. Electron dense deposits are present in the mesangium. Electron micrograph original magnification 13000X

Table 4.2   IgA Nephritis: Clinical Presentation

	(1976–1989)		(1990–1997)	
	No. of Cases	%	No. of Cases	%
1. Asymptomatic Haematuria and Proteinuria	368	65.0%	81	46%
2. Gross Haematuria	69	12.5%	7	4%
3. Nephrotic Syndrome	42	8.0%	22	13%
4. Acute Nephritis	9	2.0%	24	14%
5. Chronic Renal Failure	24	4.0%	2	1%
6. Hypertension	36	6.5%	34	19%
7. Others	–	–	6	3%
TOTAL	548	100%	176	100%

proteinuria, seldom do they develop renal failure. So they were biopsied only when proteinuria exceeded 2 gm in the 1990's. The data between 1976 and 1989 is more representative of the profile of IgA nephritis in Singapore.

Table 4.3 shows that the number of renal biopsies for patients with IgA nephritis has decreased dramatically since the adoption of the 2 gm criterion for biopsy in the 1990's as the majority of patients had mild proteinuria and our biopsies before 1990 had shown that many had mild DPGN. Interestingly, as a whole, the profile before and after 1990 has not changed very much but the data before 1990 is more representative of the profile of IgA nephritis as the number of patients are larger and they are biopsied when they had less than 2 gm of proteinuria compared to those after 1990.

2. A small proportion of patients with asymptomatic haematuria and proteinuria have Minimal Lesion which has an excellent prognosis.

3. Occasionally one may see Membranous GN and very rarely Mesangiocapillary GN. In both instances SLE has to be

Table 4.3   IgA Nephritis: Histopathology

	(1976–1989)		(1990–1997)	
	No. of Cases	%	No. of Cases	%
1. Minimal Change	11	2.0%	3	2%
2. Focal Proliferative GN	49	9.0%	23	13%
3. Diffuse Mesangial Proliferative GN	389	71.0%	126	72%
4. Focal Global Sclerosis	23	4.0%	7	4%
5. Focal & Segmental Sclerosis (FSGS)	35	6.5%	9	5%
6. Diffuse Selerosing GN	41	7.5%	6	3%
7. Others	–	–	2	1%
TOTAL	548	100%	176	100%

excluded. Full house immunoglobulins on IMF study is a clue to the diagnosis of SLE as the cause of the nephritis.

4. Focal and segmental glomerulosclerosis (FSGS) and diffuse sclerosing GN connote a bad prognosis.

Most patients with asymptomatic haematuria and proteinuria have a benign course as they are likely to have mesangial IgA nephritis which has a favourable prognosis in most cases. No treatment is required for most of these patients and all they require is reassurance. They could be followed up by their general practitioners and have their blood pressure, urine microscopy, serum creatinine and urinary protein checked once a year. It is important to treat any existing hypertension as uncontrolled hypertension often leads to renal impairment in patients with IgA nephritis.

In those patients with IgA nephritis and significant glomerulosclerosis especially in the presence of severe proteinuria, the prognosis is guarded. Patients with crescents on biopsy have a poorer long-term prognosis.

On long-term follow-up, some patients may develop gross haematuria precipitated by upper respiratory tract infections or exercise. They may have colicky loin pain due to clot colic. These patients require reassurance, rest and plenty of fluids as well as antibiotics for the respiratory tract infections.

Those who develop oedema or the nephrotic syndrome will require diuretic therapy. In those with mild diffuse mesangial proliferative GN with nephrotic syndrome, a 12-week course of prednisolone therapy starting at 60 mg/day or 1 mg/kg body weight and tailing off by 12 weeks may induce a remission in about 50% of cases. These are patients with selective proteinuria. Hypertension when it occurs must be treated aggressively as uncontrolled hypertension can lead to rapid deterioration of renal function, culminating in ESRF.

On the whole, most patients with asymptomatic haematuria and proteinuria due to IgA nephritis run a benign course, except for about 30% (usually associated with glomerulosclerosis and heavy proteinuria) who develop renal failure over a period of 10 years. These patients would ultimately require renal transplantation or dialysis. In other words, IgA nephritis is not always a benign disease, especially in Singapore where we have large numbers of people with the disease. It is therefore an important cause of ESRF.

Factors Influencing the Progression of IgA Nephritis

In a study of 151 patients with IgA nephritis in our Department,[6] 76% had stable renal function, 12% had slow deterioration of renal function and 11% progressed to end stage renal failure during a follow-up period of 65 ± 4.0 months (range 6 to 102 months). The cumulative renal survival at the end of 8 years is 82%.

Patients with IgA nephritis when they develop renal impairment run two different courses. One is a slowly progressive course over years which probably represents the natural history of deterioration in renal function due to the nephritis per se, resulting in a constant decline in renal function. The other course is a more rapid one, progressing to end stage renal failure within a few years, and where severe uncontrolled hypertension seems to be the major adverse factor.

A comparison of various factors which might have influenced the patients' clinical course showed that those with stable function had less proteinuria, crescents and a lower incidence of hypertension in contrast to patients who develop renal failure. The latter had more proteinuria, crescents and a higher incidence of hypertension. When proteinuria exceeded 2 gm, there was a higher incidence of renal failure as well as an increased incidence of crescents on renal biopsy. Heavier proteinuria seemed to be related to more severe histological lesions.

Our data showed that patients with crescents had a higher chance of developing end stage renal failure. Shirai found that patients who developed chronic renal failure at follow-up evaluation showed marked capsular adhesions, fibrocellular crescents and glomerular hyalinisation and sclerosis at the initial biopsy. Lawler believed that focal global sclerosis or capsular crescents adversely affected the course of the disease.

Hypertension[7] was present in 23% of the patients. It is a bad prognostic sign as 44% of those with hypertension developed chronic renal failure. Their histological lesions were also severe with 97% having associated glomerulosclerosis and 22% associated crescents.

The conclusion from our study was that IgA nephritis is not always a benign disease. It has a cumulative renal survival of 82% after 8 years. The data showed that renal deterioration in IgA nephritis is generally slow and progressive over a long period of time (average 7.7 years). The single most important intercurrent cause for accelerated deterioration to end stage renal failure (average 3.3 years) seems to be uncontrolled hypertension. The unfavourable long-term prognostic indices are proteinuria of more than 1 gm a day, hypertension, glomerulosclerosis exceeding 20%, presence of crescents, medial hyperplasia of blood vessels on renal biopsy. It would appear that control of hypertension is of paramount importance in preventing or delaying the onset of end stage renal failure.

How does glomerulonephritis come about?

Most forms of nephritis arise because of abnormal immunological mechanisms in the body. The immunological system defends our body against invasion by foreign organisms (bacteria, viruses, fungi, parasites). It does so by mobilising a certain group of white corpuscles called lymphocytes to attack and destroy the foreign organism. It can also cause these lymphocytes to produce antibodies which are directed against the foreign organism. To be specific, the antibodies are directed against the antigen on the surface of the organism. During this warfare, the antibody reacts with the antigen to form clumps or complexes (antigen-antibody complexes) and these circulate in the bloodstream.

As the blood containing these immune complexes passes through the body, the complexes are deposited in the glomeruli of the kidneys since the glomeruli filter all our blood. In the glomeruli an inflammatory reaction is triggered off and spreads to other glomeruli. This inflammation of the glomerulus leads to leakage of red blood cells and protein into the urine, hence explaining the presence of red blood cells and protein as an abnormal finding in patients suffering from glomerulonephritis. If the inflammatory reaction is temporary then the damage is negligible and healing occurs rapidly. If the inflammation continues, sometimes for years, more and more glomeruli become damaged. With time, the glomeruli die and appear as sclerosis in a renal biopsy. When sclerosis becomes severe (diffuse sclerosing GN) renal failure occurs.

The above is a relatively simplistic explanation for what is in fact a very complex orchestrated chain of inflammatory reactions which take place. In addition to the lymphocytes, other types of white corpuscles, platelets, clotting factors which induce a low grade intravascular coagulation and other forms of acute and chronic phase reactants including cytokines also take part in the inflammation.

We do not know why some people develop glomerulonephritis and others do not or why some have a mild disease while others develop renal failure. Research is being conducted here and abroad. One of the beliefs is that certain individuals have the ability to clear these antigen antibody complexes very rapidly and thus avoid nephritis. Others may have some deficiency in one or several aspects of the immune system resulting in poor clearance of the complexes and therefore develop nephritis.

Renal Biopsy

This is a procedure which enables the kidney specialist to obtain a sample of kidney tissue in order to determine the particular type of kidney disease the patient has. The patient is admitted into hospital. After the procedure he stays overnight and if there is no blood in the urine the next day the patient can be discharged.

For renal biopsy, the position of the kidney is first localised by means of intravenous pyelogram or ultrasound examination of the kidney. The patient lies prone on his or her abdomen and the position of the kidney is marked on the back. Local anaesthetic is administered to the skin down to the surface of the kidney. The biopsy needle is then introduced into the kidney and a core of kidney tissue taken out, usually about 1 mm wide and 10 to 20 mm long. The patient should feel no pain and after the biopsy he rests in bed until the next day. He is encouraged to drink about 3 litres of fluid to wash out the blood leaking from the puncture wound in the kidney. A few patients may pass blood in the urine but this will usually go off.

The sample of kidney tissue is sent for light microscopy, immunofluorescence and electron microscopic examination. This will give a clue to the nature, type and severity of the kidney disease. It will therefore be of use for prognosis and planning of management of the renal disease.

What investigations are usually performed on a patient who is suspected of having Glomerulonephritis?

A fresh specimen of urine is examined for protein, red cells and casts. Nowadays, by using a phase contrast microscope, the type of red cells in the urine can be further characterised as to their site of origin. Red cells resulting from glomerulonephritis are usually distorted (dysmorphic) whereas those arising from some other source of non-glomerular bleeding (stone, tumour) are usually of normal shape (isomorphic).

Blood samples are taken to determine the level of creatinine to assess renal function. A 24-hour urine collection is usually requested for the estimation of creatinine clearance and protein loss in the urine. Further samples of blood are sent to exclude or confirm the diagnosis of various forms of kidney diseases, especially SLE causing lupus nephritis.

If it is decided after the above tests that the patient will require a renal biopsy then an intravenous pyelogram may be ordered prior to the renal biopsy. If the biopsy is to be performed under ultrasound guidance an IVP is usually not necessary.

Significance of Repeatedly Passing Blood in the Urine (Visible Blood or Gross Haematuria)

The repeated passing of red or brown urine, an indication of the presence of blood in the urine especially if associated with fever or sore throat or other respiratory tract infection, is likely to be a symptom of glomerulonephritis. Further examination may reveal that the patient is also passing protein in the urine. A kidney biopsy in these patients will usually show a particular type of glomerulonephritis called IgA nephritis. IgA means immunoglobulin A. The disease is so named because when the kidney biopsy specimen is examined under a special immunofluorescent technique, it stains strongly for IgA.

There are of course other causes for passing grossly blood-stained urine, one of which is a condition called stress haematuria. This occurs in some people after they have engaged in heavy exercise or after jogging for a few kilometres. The condition is due to trauma of blood vessels in the urinary bladder. The best way to confirm the diagnosis is to pass a tube called a cystoscope into the bladder and identify the source of the bleeding. Sometimes kidney stones or even a tumour in the bladder can also cause gross bleeding into the urine on exertion. If in doubt it is always wise to have an IVP to exclude a stone and a cystoscopy to exclude a tumour.

Significance of finding a small amount of blood and protein in the urine on routine medical examination

The medical term for this is asymptomatic haematuria and proteinuria. Many forms of glomerulonephritis present in this way with the patient well and healthy with absolutely no symptoms. In fact some patients start to experience symptoms after they have been told they have kidney disease. They become neurotic and require a lot of reassurance that this type of kidney condition does not cause backache.

Asymptomatic haematuria is usually discovered following pre-employment or life assurance screening. Such patients will need a microscopic examination of the urine, blood tests and 24-hour urine collection for creatinine clearance and protein estimation. Those found to have more severe abnormalities will require a renal biopsy. In the Singapore context, the majority of these patients will have IgA nephritis.

We shall first deal with those who have gross bleeding in the urine. If there is no accompanying loss of protein in the urine the outlook is good, though the presence of blood in the urine is alarming. The bleeding will clear up after one to two days but may return whenever the patient has fever or a sore throat. If he has a throat infection, he may require antibiotics. He should drink plenty of fluids to dilute the blood in the urine so that it can pass out easily without clotting and causing a clot colic. He should, of course, try to rest and refrain from heavy work. With the passage of years the episodes of bleeding will gradually disappear.

In patients with more than 1 gm of protein loss in the urine the disease is more severe whether it is in a patient with gross bleeding or in one who has asymptomatic haematuria and proteinuria. A renal biopsy will usually show some scars and with time some will develop hypertension and renal failure.

It is a good policy to remind patients even with mild urinary abnormalities to see their general practitioner once a year to have the urine, serum creatinine and urinary protein as well as blood pressure checked as there will always be some patients with mild urinary abnormalities who may develop hypertension or have progression of their disease with worsening proteinuria. In such cases it is important that their blood pressure be controlled and renal biopsy performed to assess the renal status.

REFERENCES

1. Glassock RJ, Adler SG, Ward HJ, Cohen AH: Primary Glomerular Diseases. In: Brenner BM, Rector FC, eds. The Kidney. Philadelphia: WB Saunders Company, 1991, 1182–1279.

2. Potter EV, Lipschultz SA, Abidh S et al: Twelve to seventeen year follow up of patients with poststreptococcal acute glomerulonephritis in Trinidad. *New Engl J Med.* 1982, **307**:725–729.

3. Drachman R, Aladjem M, Vardy PA: Natural History of an acute glomerulonephritis epidemic in children: An 11 to 12 year follow up. *Israel J Med Sci.* 1982, **18**:603–607.

4. Singhal PC, Malik GH, Narayan G, Khan AS, Bhusnurmath S, Datta BN, Chugh KS: Prognosis of Post-Streptococcal Glomerulonephritis: Chandigarh Study. *Ann Acad Med*, Singapore, 1982, **11**:36–41.

5. Kincaid-Smith P: Severe acute oliguric renal failure in glomerular and vascular disease. In: Kincaid-Smith P. The Kidney: A clinico-pathological study. Oxford: Blackwell Scientific Publications, 1975, 259–275.

6. Woo KT, Edmondson RPS, Wu AYT, Chiang GSC, Pwee HS, Lim CH: The Natural History of IgA Nephritis in Singapore. *Clin Nephrol.* 1986, **25**:15–21.

7. Woo KT, Wong KS, Lau YK, GSC Chiang, CH Lim : Hypertension in IgA Nephropathy. *Ann Acad Med,* Singapore, 1988, **17**:583–588.

CHAPTER 5

Nephrotic Syndrome

Nephrotic Syndrome is a clinical entity of multiple causes characterised by increased glomerular permeability manifested by massive proteinuria of more than 3 gm per day associated with oedema and hypoalbuminaemia of less than 30 gm. Very often, there is also associated hypercholesterolaemia and hypertriglyceridaemia and lipiduria. Any glomerular lesion may be associated, at least temporarily, with heavy proteinuria in the nephrotic range.

Table 5.1 shows the histological distribution of Primary Nephrotic Syndrome occurring in Singapore. As long as a patient presents with the Nephrotic Syndrome he would be offerred a renal biopsy. The 2 gm criterion would not have affected the biopsy rate of this group of patients. Therefore the data before and after 1990 are comparable. In the 1990's, Mesangial Proliferative GN is no longer the commonest form of Nephrotic Syndrome seen. Minimal Change Disease is the commonest and this appears unique. If we combine Minimal Change with Focal Global Sclerosis what it means is that 49% of Adult Nephrotics in Singapore are likely to respond to Prednisolone or Cyclophosphamide.

In many Western countries, Membranous GN is the commonest GN, accounting for about 35%. In Asian countries, Mesangial Proliferative GN is the commonest (as was Singapore before the 1990's). The high incidence of Mesangial Proliferative GN was attributed to infection in these countries. IgA nephritis with Mesangial Proliferative GN is an uncommon cause of the Nephrotic Syndrome, accounting for about 8% of Nephrotics. However we are now seeing more patients with Minimal Change and Focal Global Sclerosis not responding to Steroids or Prednisolone, meaning that they have Focal and Segmental Glomerulosclerosis (FSGS) which is less responsive to therapy. What this implies is that the true incidence of FSGS is not at 12% but is probably closer to 15% or more. In other words, there is a rising incidence of FSGS in keeping with the incidence in other countries.[1] The incidence of Membranous GN remains the same (about 10%). Mesangio-Capillary GN (MCGN) and Crescenteric GN are uncommon. About 20 years ago MCGN was common in the West and it was related to infection, now it is uncommon.

The epidemiology of GN follows a racial and geographical distribution which is influenced by the environment (infection) and the foodstuff we ingest (allergens) or the air we breathe in and this may be the explanation for why taxi-drivers in Singapore seem to thave a higher incidence of GN (personal observation).

Table 5.1 Nephrotic Syndrome in Singapore

	(1976–1989)		(1990–1997)	
	No. of Cases	%	No. of Cases	%
1. Minimal Change	95	22%	49	30%
2. Focal Global Sclerosis	74	17%	31	19%
3. Mesangial Proliferative GN	158	37%	43	25%
4. Focal & Segmental Sclerosing (FSGS)	50	12%	20	12%
5. Membranous GN	40	9%	16	10%
6. Crescenteric GN	4	1%	2	1%
7. Diffuse Sclerosing GN	10	2%	1	1%
8. Others	–	–	4	2%
TOTAL	431	100%	166	100%

1. MINIMAL CHANGE DISEASE

This is also referred to as Lipoid Nephrosis. The renal biopsy shows normal findings on light microscopy (LM) (Fig. 5.1), but there is foot process fusion on electron microscopy (EM) (Fig. 5.2). Immunofluorescence (IMF) studies may show IgE but usually there is no immunoglobulin staining on IMF.

Young children are especially affected with a peak from 2 to 4 years. Minimal Change accounts for 60 to 70% of all idiopathic nephrotic syndrome in children and 10 to 30% in adults. In Singapore this is also the commonest lesion in adults (30%). Hypertension and renal impairment are uncommon complications and microscopic haematuria is rare. Shaloub[2] considers this disease a disorder in T cell function with abnormal lymphokine production. Focal Global Sclerosis (FGS) accounts for 19% of Nephrotics in adults in Singapore. Clinically FGS behaves like Minimal Change, is steroid responsive and has a good prognosis.

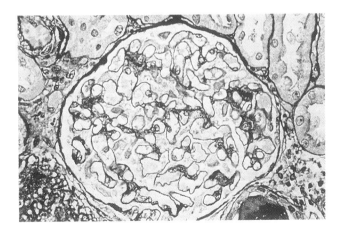

Fig. 5.1   Minimal lesion. The glomerulus is normal on light microscopy. PAS Stain original magnification 400X

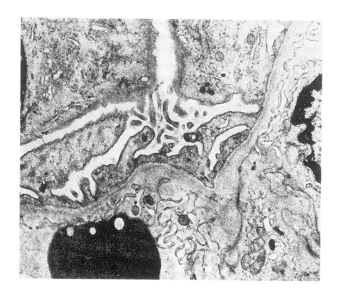

Fig. 5.2   Fusion of foot processes is seen along the glomerular basement membrane. Electron micrograph original magnification 13000X

Treatment consists of a three months' course of prednisolone. In those who fail to respond or where they have frequent relapses, cyclophosphamide for three months may induce long lasting remissions.

This is a disease with a good prognosis even though the relapse rates are high. Depending on a patient's response to prednisolone and his frequency of relapses various categories have been described. Thirty eight per cent are primary responders, non-relapsers. If a patient has less than 2 relapses in the first 6 months of the initial response he is a primary responder, infrequent relapser (19%). If he had 2 or more relapses in 6 months he is a primary responder, frequent relapser (42%). Five per cent of patients do not respond to steroids following an initial response (secondary non-responder).[3]

If there is no response to initial treatment but response after completion of treatment the patient is said to be a primary non-responder, late responder (7%). A continuing non-responder shows no response at any time (30% of primary non-responders). Spontaneous remission without treatment refers to the group of spontaneous responders. Relapse may occur after treatment is withdrawn or during reduction of steroids (steroid dependent responder).

White[4] reported lasting remission in 7% and Habib[5] in 18% of patients. Arneil[6] found that 40% were free of disease 5 to 10 years after a single course with no relapse. The frequency of relapse decreases after 10 years.

In a study among adults, Cameron[7] showed that 18% responded with early loss of proteinuria but 70% of them relapsed, 63% repeatedly. A small number, after repeated relapse and remission acquired steroid unresponsiveness. They displayed focal glomerulosclerosis on renal biopsy. The use of cytotoxics is recommended in this group. Fifty to 60% of adults with Minimal Lesion will remit for 5 years or more. Those who fail to respond to Cyclophosphamide can be given a course of Cyclosporine A.

Of 49 adults followed up by Cameron for 19 years, 9 had died but only one from uraemia and 3 from complications of treatment. Twenty-nine of the original 49 were well and on no treatment. In Habib's series,[8] 14 of 209 followed up from 1 to 10 years had died, only 3 from CRF 5 to 8 years from onset (steroid resistant). The survival rates in Cameron's series was 98% at 5 years and 97% at 10 years.

A patient with Minimal Lesion has an excellent long-term prognosis if he has minimal glomerular lesion on light microscopy, foot process fusion on electron microscopy, absence of immunoglobulins on immunofluorescence (IMF), and complete remission following a course of steroids. Even so, multiple relapses will still occur.

2. FOCAL AND SEGMENTAL GLOMERULO SCLEROSIS (FSGS) (Fig. 5.3)

Rich in 1957 first described focal sclerosis of the glomeruli especially at the juxtamedullary zones of the cortex. The disease is due to an Abnormal T cell function with lymphokine inducing a proteinuric factor.

There is a slight preponderance of males with a peak at 20 to 30 years accounting for 10 to 20% of idiopathic nephrotic syndrome. The incidence of FSGS is rising in most countries.[1] In Singapore it is now about 15%.

About 70–90% present as the Nephrotic Syndrome; hypertension may be an associated feature.

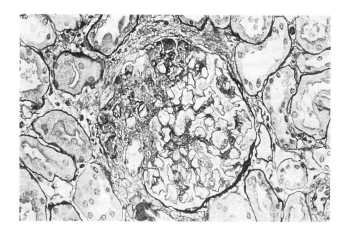

Fig. 5.3   Focal segmental sclerosis. A segment of the glomerulus is sclerotic. PAS Stain original magnification 300X

Light microscopy shows segmental hyaline sclerosis with an increase in mesangial matrix, spreading from the hilus with no proliferation or necrosis. There is subsequent progression to global sclerosis. EM shows foot process fusion with subendothelial and mesangial electron dense deposits and sclerosis. IMF shows IgM and C3 staining.

The majority of patients with this form of nephritis experience a progressive decline in GFR; hypertension and persistent proteinuria. Initially patients present with asymptomatic proteinuria but often they ultimately become nephrotic. Initial studies reported little benefit with treatment. Nowadays with treatment, response range from 30% to 50% (include partial response). High dose Prednisolone (1 mg/kg BW a day) for first 2 months, then 30 mg for 3rd month and thereafter reduce gradually to 10 mg and maintain till end of 6 months. Those who do not respond to prednisolone should have Cyclosphosphamide at 2 mg/kg BW a day together with Prednisolone (30 mg/day) for 3 months, then reduce and maintain for another 3 months. In those who fail Cyclophosphamide they could be given Cyclosporine A at 5 mg/kg BW a day for 3 months, than 4 mg at 4th month, then 3 mg at 5th month and 2 mg at 6th month and maintain for 1 year. There may be a potential role for FK 506 (0.1 to 0.2 mg/kg BW a day).

The 5-year and 10-year survival according to Cameron's series[7] are 70% and 50% respectively. The presence of nephrotic syndrome affects the prognosis. Beaufils[9] reported a 90% 10-year survival in non-nephrotic patients and a 45% survival in those who were nephrotic.

Rydel et al[10] reported a renal survival at 10 years for 100% of responders, 39% for non-responders and 47% for untreated nephrotics while Banfi[11] reported survival of 98% for responders and 30% for non-responders.

Thirty per cent of renal allografts in patients with FSGS as the original disease experience a recurrence of the disease. Pregnant patients with FSGS do poorly as there is a high incidence of pre-eclampsia and renal impairment.

Among children with this disease, 30 to 40% respond to steroids. If FSGS develops later on a background of Minimal Change Lesion, patients remain steroid responsive. However if FSGS develops on a background of Mesangial Proliferative Lesion, the prognosis is poorer.

3. MESANGIAL PROLIFERATIVE GLOMERULONEPHRITIS (Fig. 5.4)

Histologically there is increase in mesangial cells and matrix with no capillary wall thickening. IMF is negative staining in the majority (44%) whilst others shown IgM, IgA either predominantly or with other Ig in equal or lesser strength. In those with negative IMF the EM also show no electron dense deposits (EDD).

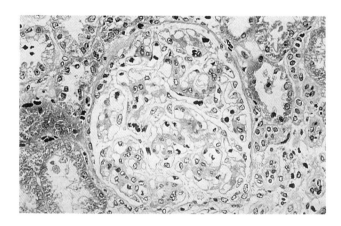

Fig. 5.4 Mesangial proliferative glomerulonephritis. The glomerulus shows an increase in mesangial matrix and cells. HE Stain original magnification 300X

It occurs in about 25% of idiopathic nephrotic syndrome among adults in Singapore but appears to be a much less common cause of nephrotic syndrome in Western countries. IgA nephritis accounts for about 8% of nephrotic syndrome seen in Singapore and is therefore an uncommon cause of nephrotic syndrome. (Biopsy data before 1990 are more representative as the numbers for IgA nephritis are larger).

The long-term evolution of this type of nephritis is not well understood. This discussion excludes IgA nephritis which has been dealt with earlier but it includes IgM nephropathy, IgG and the IMF negative group.

Patients with this lesion who become nephrotic and develop focal and segmental sclerosis have a higher incidence of developing chronic renal failure (CRF). About 30% of those with nephrotic syndrome experience complete remissions with steroid. They are usually the ones with mild mesangial proliferation with no focal and segmental sclerosis.

In those patients therefore who have mild proliferation of the mesangium with no evidence of focal and segmental sclerosis and negative immunoglobulin staining on IMF, a trial of steroid therapy should be offered as they have a good chance of achieving remission. Habib[8] in fact considered such patients as part of the spectrum of Minimal Change GN. Waldher[12] reported that more than 50% of patients with Mesangial Proliferative GN were steroid resistant, 70% with associated focal and segmental sclerosis. There is a need for controlled therapeutic trials in patients with this form of nephritis. In our experience those with selective proteinuria tend to respond to steroids and failing that cyclophosphamide. Those who fail cyclophosphamide can be offerred Cyclosporine A.

4. MEMBRANOUS GLOMERULONEPHRITIS (Figs. 5.5 and 5.6)

Patients with Membranous Glomerulonephritis usually present as Nephrotic Syndrome. Characteristically there is thickening of glomerular capillary wall on LM. EM shows electron dense deposits (EDD) in a subepithelial location. IMF shows linear "granular" IgG. Majority of patients are above 40 years of age at diagnosis with a peak around 40 to 50 years. Males are more commonly affected than females. This is the commonest GN in the West constituting 35% of all nephrotic syndrome but in Singapore it is present in about 10% of all idiopathic nephrotic syndrome.

Hypertension and azotaemia are late features of the disease. Microscopic haematuria is common but gross haematuria is a rare feature. Renal vein thrombosis is secondary to the glomerulopathy rather than the cause of it.

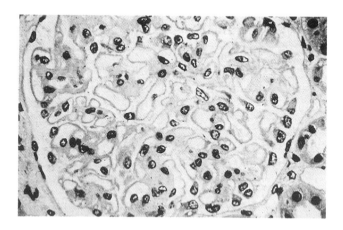

Fig. 5.5   Membranous glomerulonephritis. There is diffuse thickening of the glomerular basement membrane. HE Stain original magnification 500X

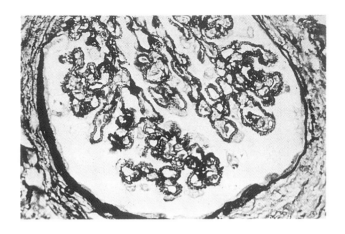

Fig. 5.6 Membranous glomerulonephritis. Well formed spikes are seen along the glomerular basement membrane using the silver stain. PAAg-MT Stain original magnification 400X

This disease runs an indolent and slowly progressive course with remissions and exacerbations of the nephrotic syndrome. Children have a better prognosis with less than 5% CRF after 5 years and a 90% 10year survival. Adults however have a less benign course; 25% achieve spontaneous remission with another 25% spontaneous partial remission (less than 2 gm proteinuria). Cameron's series[13] had a 75% 5-year and 50% 10-year survival. Even patients with partial remission have a better outlook than those who have no response at all.

In a patient with Membranous GN who develops progressive renal failure within a few months, the following should be considered:

1. Hypersensitivity interstitial nephritis
2. Superimposed crescents
3. Renal vein thrombosis
4. Profound hypovolaemia from proteinuria

A controlled trial with high dose alternate-day prednisolone in the USA has reported a reduction in proteinuria and progression of CRF.[14] However, if there is already abnormal GFR, steroid therapy is not of much use. We would offer a 3 months course of prednisolone therapy and failing that cyclophosphamide. There is a potential role for other agents like Chlorambucil (0.15–0.2 mg/kg BW/day),[23] Cyclosporine A (5 mg/kg BW/day) and FK 506 (0.1–0.2 mg/kg BW/day).[24]

5. MESANGIOCAPILLARY GLOMERULONEPHRITIS (MCGN) (Fig. 5.7)

The presence of prominent increase in mesangial cellularity and their extension into peripheral capillary wall leads to the appearance of thickened and reduplicated capillary wall on LM. EM of Type I MCGN shows electron dense subendothelial deposits. In Type II MCGN or what is referred to as Dense Deposit Disease (DDD), EDD is found within the substance of the glomerular basement membrane proper. IMF of Type I shows

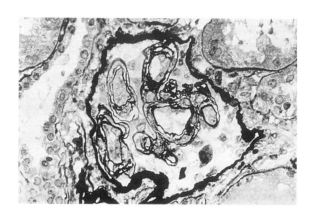

Fig. 5.7 Mesangiocapillary glomerulonephritis. A double contour glomerular basement membrane is seen. PAAg-MT Stain original magnification 500X

irregular C3 in a granular distribution along the capillary walls with IgG and/or IgM in about 50%. In Type II MCGN only C3 is found in the mesangium.

Complement: In Type I MCGN, 70% have prolonged depression of C3. C1q and C4 may be low when C3 is low. In Type II MCGN there is persistent low C3 (persistent hypocomplementemic GN). C3Nef, a gamma-globulin that cleaves C3 is also present. The values of C1q and C4 are normal.

All age groups are involved, especially those aged 5 to 15 years. It occurs in 5 to 10% of children with the nephrotic syndrome. Fifty per cent have associated upper respiratory tract infection and 40% have high anti-streptolysin 0 titre (ASOT).

Half of patients with MCGN present as the nephrotic syndrome, 30% as asymptomatic haematuria and proteinuria, and the remaining 20% as acute nephritic syndrome. Hypertension is present in 33%. About 50% develop renal impairment. If the patient is nephrotic and crescents are present on renal biopsy the prognosis is worse. Idiopathic MCGN occurs uncommonly in Singapore.

This type of nephritis has a relentless but slowly progressive course. The bad prognostic features are low GFR, hypertension, persistent nephrotic syndrome and the presence of diffuse crescents on renal biopsy.

For Type I MCGN (Subendothelial Deposits) the 5-year and 10-year survival are 80% and 60% respectively. For Type II MCGN (Dense Deposit Disease) the respective survival rates are poorer, 60% and 45% at 5 and 10 years. Other series reported a poorer prognosis in the presence of nephrotic syndrome with 40% survival at 10 years, compared to 85% at 10 years for patients with no nephrotic syndrome.

But even in the patients with nephrotic syndrome the occasional remission has been reported. In general, however, those with Type II disease have a poorer outlook.

For the moment there is no clearly established form of treatment. McEnery[15] reported the beneficial effects of continuous low dose prednisolone whereas Kincaid-Smith[16] reported 3-year survival of 82% using a combination regimen of cyclophosphamide, persantin and warfarin (Melbourne Cocktail) in an uncontrolled trial. We would advocate a 3 months course of prednisolone and failing that cyclophosphamide.

6. HEREDITARY NEPHRITIS AND DEAFNESS (ALPORT'S SYNDROME)

This is often discovered in childhood or young adult life. Males are affected in an autosomal dominant fashion.

Patients have gross or recurrent microscopic haematuria which is worsened by respiratory infections. Some may have occasional loin pain.

Sensory neural deafness (high frequency sound) occurs in 30 to 50% and is usually associated with thrombocytopathia. Ocular features are also present in the form of spherophakia, lenticonus, myopia, retinitis pigmentosa and amaurosis.

Renal failure is usual before 40 years.

Pathology

Light microscopy shows endocapillary proliferation which is focal or diffuse associated with focal sclerosis and tubulo-interstitial lesions with presence of foam cells. Electron microscopy shows irregularly thickened and attenuated basement membrane with pronounced splitting and lamination of the lamina densa. The splits enclose electron-lucent areas. Immunofluorescence studies usually show negative staining with occasional C3.

This condition is due to a disorder of basement membrane synthesis involving the X chromosome with a defect in the structural gene.

The course is one of slowly progressive renal failure.

CLINICAL ASPECTS OF THE NEPHROTIC SYNDROME

The term "Syndrome" implies "A Symptom Complex". It comprises:

1. Oedema
2. Proteinuria of 3 gm or more
3. Hypoproteinaemia, ie. serum albumin of less than 30 gm
4. Hypercholesterolaemia is often an associated feature.

Oedema

i. The degree of oedema is proportional to the serum albumin concentration.
ii. Reduction of plasma oncotic pressure leads to a reduction in plasma volume (20 to 30%).
iii. Hypovolaemia stimulates renin which in turn causes aldosteronism with resulting Na^+ retention and K^+ excretion.
iv. When oedema fluid accumulates, the urine Na^+ may be nil (normal is 80 to 150 mEq/day).

Renal Function

1. The kidney excretes urea and creatinine normally but retains Na^+. There is increased excretion of K^+ and protein.
2. Blood urea alone as a test of renal function is falsely low as patients are in negative nitrogen balance.
3. Pre-renal failure may occur because of glomerular hypoperfusion.

Symptoms

1. Frothy urine accompanies proteinuria.
2. Patients complain that their legs are heavy, swollen, cold and numb.
3. They feel lethargic and tired because of negative nitrogen balance and anaemia.
4. Anorexia and diarrhoea may result from oedema of the gut.

SIGNS OF NEPHROTIC SYNDROME

1. Oedema may be present periorbitally, in the abdominal wall, genitalia, knee joints, ascites, pleural effusion, conjunctival oedema and retinal oedema. Long standing oedema causes pale striae in the distended skin.
2. Pallor may simulate anaemia. The nephrotic facies is often characteristic.
3. Muscle wasting is due to loss of skeletal muscle. In addition, steroid therapy causes proximal myopathy.
4. Nails may show transverse white bands called Muerchke's Bands due to low serum albumin.
5. Hypertension if it is due to nephritis may augur badly for the patients as it usually indicates a more severe histological lesion. Steroids too can cause hypertension.

Infections

1. Pneumococcal peritonitis is a well-known complication of the nephrotic syndrome.
2. Patients are prone to lung and skin infections.
3. In the Nephrotic Crisis the patient presents with severe abdominal pain with vomiting and tenderness. At laparotomy sterile fluid with fibrin strands is found. The differential diagnosis for this condition includes primary peritonitis, perforated appendicitis, perforated gastric ulcer and "cramps" due to excess diuretics.

COMPLICATIONS OF NEPHROTIC SYNDROME

1. Subnutritional state.
2. Infections.
3. Clotting tendency due to increased clotting factors (V, VIII, Fibrinogen), increased platelet aggregation and low anti-thrombin III. This leads to spontaneous thrombosis involving veins and arteries.
4. Atheroma formation giving rise to ischaemic heart disease and renal artery stenosis and renal vein thrombosis.
5. Hypovolaemic collapse.
6. Complications of treatment, eg. side effects of steroids and cytotoxic drugs.

CAUSES OF NEPHROTIC SYNDROME

— 80% due to glomerulonephritis
— 20% due to miscellaneous causes

1. Diabetes mellitus
2. Amyloidosis

3. Precipitating causes of renal vein thrombosis (RVT)
   i. Nephrotic syndrome (hypercoagulable state)
   ii. Renal amyloid gives rise to thrombosis of intrarenal veins
   iii. Hypernephroma gives rise to obstruction and RVT
   iv. Trauma of renal veins
   v. Severe dehydration especially in infants suffering from gastroenteritis

   RVT is a complication of Nephrotic Syndrome and not a cause of Nephrotic Syndrome

4. Malignancy: Hodgkin's Disease, bronchogenic carcinoma, cancer of the breast, bowel, leukaemias, myeloma.
5. Infections: Hepatitis B and C, Malaria, syphilis, leprosy.
6. Drugs: Trimethadione, penicillamine, phenindione, gold, mercury, bismuth, captopril, NSAIDS.
7. Autoimmune Disease, SLE, Cryoglobulinemia, Thyrotoxicosis.
8. Congenital Nephrotic Syndrome
   Causes: Congenital syphilis, cytomegalovirus infection, mercury poisoning, maternal tuberculosis.
9. Miscellaneous: Prophylactic inoculation (smallpox, polio, tetanus), bee stings, pollen allergy.

MANAGEMENT OF NEPHROTIC SYNDROME

I. General Treatment

1. Diuretic Treatment
   These are the major agents in treatment:
   i. Frusemide can be used alone. Increase the dose till diuresis occurs. K^+ supplements are required.
   ii. Spironolactone should be avoided if serum K^+ is high or patient has renal impairment.
   iii. Chlortride has a synergistic action with frusemide and spironolactone.

   We usually use a combination regimen of all 3 diuretics as they have synergistic actions (see chapter on Diuretics).

2. Treatment of hypertension.

3. Treatment of infections. Use the appropriate antibiotics.

4. Diet: The patient requires a high protein, low salt diet with fluid restriction.

5. Infusion of Na^+ free albumin induces diuresis but its benefit is evanescent.

6. Use ACE inhibitor or Angiotensin II Receptor Antagonist (ATRA) to reduce GFR and limit protein loss in urine.

II. Specific Treatment

1. Investigate and try to elucidate the cause of Nephrotic Syndrome and if possible remove or treat it.

2. Check through list of causes and investigate accordingly. In all patients always exclude SLE.

Do anti-nuclear factor (ANF), anti-DNA, and serum complement. A patient with membranous glomerulonephritis should be screened for hepatitis B antigen and antibody.

III. Treatment with Steroids and Cytotoxic Agents

Primary Treatment to induce remission.

1. Minimal change GN and lupus nephritis respond well to a course of prednisolone starting at 60 mg or 1 mg/kg BW/day and reducing gradually over a period of 3 months. For those who fail to respond to prednisolone or who are frequent relapsers, cyclophosphamide (2 mg/kg BW) for 3 months is advocated. Those who fail cyclophosphamide

can be given a course of Cyclosporine A at 5 mg/kg BW for 3 months with reduction over the next 3 months and maintain at 2 mg/kg BW up to a year.

2. Mild diffuse mesangial proliferative GN may respond to prednisolone, failing that try cyclophosphamide.

3. Membranous GN may respond to a course of prednisolone for a period of 3 months, failing that try cyclophosphamide.

4. Focal and Segmental Glomerulosclerosis may respond to Prednisolone and Cyclophosphamide for 6 months. If no response, try Cyclosporine.

5. Other newer agents include FK 506 (0.1–0.2 mg/kg BW/day)[24] and Mycophenolate Mofetil (MMF) (0.75–1 gm twice daily)[25] for 3 months.

IV. Persantin and Warfarin Plus Regimen (P and W + regimen)

All patients who fail to respond to Steroids and Cytotoxics should be offerred P and W + regimen which would help to retard progression to ESRF.

1. Persantin (Dipyridamole) — anti-platelet and anti-PDGF, 75 to 100 mg tds with low dose Warfarin (anti-thrombotic), 1 to 3 mg (INR < 1.6)
2. Treat Hypertension
3. ACE Inhibitor to reduce intra-glomerular Hypertension
4. Angiotensin Receptor Antagonist (ATRA) to reduce intra-glomerular Hypertension (Losartan)
5. Restricted Protein Diet (0.8 gm/kg BW) to decrease afferent arteriolar vasodilation
6. Treat High Lipids as Cholesterol is toxic to mesangial cells

Therapeutic Concepts of Proteinuria and Intra-Glomerular Hypertension

Proteinuria is the hallmark of renal disease.[17] Proteinuria can also be used as a prognostic marker. In patients with glomerulonephritis, those with more than 1 gram of protein excretion per day in the urine are more likely to have glomerulosclerosis or scarring of the kidneys on renal biopsy and those exceeding 2 grams a day a higher incidence of developing renal failure on long term follow up.[18] Hitherto if was believed that proteinuria is the result of damage to the kidneys but recently, evidence suggest that the converse is also true, that proteinuria can also directly cause renal damage.

When there is excessive leakage of protein in the renal tubules, the proximal tubular cells (PTC) become overloaded with protein. Lysosomes present in the PTC when they engulf excessive proteins would swell and rupture and release injurious lysosomal enzymes which cause tubulointerstitial damage and fibrosis and with time give rise to renal failure. In the second mechanism, protein overload of the PTC also triggers the release of certain growth factors such as platelet-derived growth factor (PDGF) and transforming growth factor-beta (TGF-β) which are mitogenic to the PTC. They cause excessive production of collagen as well as interstitial cell proliferation eventually leading to fibrosis and renal failure. Finally, protein overloading of the PTC causes the activation of transcriptase genes which in turn trigger genes encoding vasoactive and inflammatory mediators, the release of these lead to vasoconstriction and inflammation of the renal tissue with injury and renal failure.[19]

Therapeutic reduction of proteinuria in kidney disease is now considered as important as the reduction of BP in hypertensive patients as both are important in the preservation of renal function. Normally the two kidneys in our body excrete less than 150 mg of protein in the urine a day. We must try to reduce proteinuria to as low a level in our patients, if possible to a level below 0.5 gram a day. One of the best strategies to protect the kidneys against damage due to proteinuria is the use of Angiotensin Converting Enzyme Inhibitor (ACEI).[20] In many renal conditions associated with proteinuria there exists a phenomenon known as Glomerular Hyperfiltration (HF)[21] which induces proteinuria apart from the direct immunological effect of the glomerulonephritis (GN) which also causes renal damage with leakage of protein into the urine. HF is a condition which occurs whenever some of the glomeruli are diseased or sclerosed. The surrounding glomeruli which are normal are then subject to excessive blood flow with vasodilatation of the afferent glomerular arteriole. In the efferent glomerular arteriole there is associated Angiotensin II (ATII) mediated vasoconstriction. Therefore with increase in blood flow at the inlet and reduction of blood flow at the outlet there is excessive amount of blood in the glomeruli which is subject to HF with the result that there is raised intraglomerular (IG) blood pressure or IG HPT. IG HPT is associated initially with increase in single nephron Glomerular Filtration Rate (GFR) with leakage of protein in the urine. With time as a consequence of IG HPT there is renal damage with glomerular sclerosis and eventually renal failure. ACEI by inhibiting the action of ATII on the efferent glomerular arteriole will cause vasodilatation thereby reducing IG HPT and preserving renal function of the affected glomeruli. About 20 to 30% of our patients given ACEI develop the side effect of a dry irritating cough which is further aggravated whenever they have a respiratory tract infection. For these patients we recommend an Angiotensin II Receptor Antagonist (ATRA) (Losartan) which does not have the side effect of cough. ATRA competes with the receptor for angiotensin and therefore inhibits the action of angiotensin. It is as effective as ACEI in the reduction of proteinuria and preservation of renal function. When using an ACEI or ATRA one should initially target for a 50% reduction of proteinuria with eventual reduction to < 0.5 gm proteinuria a day. In other words, the dose of ACEI or ATRA should be increased gradually if necessary to its maximum dose for effective reduction of proteinuria.

Salt restriction is important. For those who cannot restrict salt, 12.5 mg of hydrochlorothiazide daily can potentiate the effect of ATRA.

In summary, recent studies have highlighted the important contribution of filtered urinary protein to deterioration of renal function. In depth analysis of proteinuria may assess the degree of glomerular and tubular involvement and help in prognostication of an individual patient with proteinuria. One should consider not only the quantity but also the quality of the urinary protein. This is especially so if there is presence of significant amounts of low molecular weight (LMW) proteins in the urine. In this respect, Woo *et al*[22] reported that the presence of LMW proteins in the proteinuric SDS-PAGE patterns of patients with IgA nephritis was significantly associated with higher rates of chronic renal failure after 6 years of follow up. There was a significant correlation between the LMW patterns and tubular atrophy and tubulointerstitial lesions. This work has since been confirmed by other workers and today the presence of LMW proteinuria has been established as an adverse prognostic factor.

REFERENCES

1. Haas M, Spargo BH, Conventry S. Increasing incidence of focal-segmental glomerulosclerosis among adult nephropathies: A 20-year renal biopsy study. *Am J Kidney Dis*. 1995, **26**:740–750.

2. Shalhoub RJ. Pathogenesis of lipoid nephrosis: A disorder of T cell function. *Lancet* 1974, **2**:556–560.

3. Cameron JS. The long-term outcome of glomerular diseases. In Diseases of the kidney, (2nd edn), (ed. RN Schrier and CW Gottschalk). Little Brown, Boston 1992, 1895–1958.

4. White RHR, Glasgow EF, Mills RJ: Clinicopathological syndrome in children. *Lancet* 1970, 1:1353–1359.

5. Habib R, Kleinknecht C, Gubler MD: The Nephrotic Syndrome. In: Royer P, Mathieu H, Broyer M, Walsh A, eds. Paediatric Nephrology. Philadelphia, W B Saunders Company, 1974, 258.

6. Arneil GC, Lam C: Long term assessment of steroid therapy in childhood nephrosis. *Lancet* 1966, 2:819–821.

7. Cameron JS: The problem of focal segmental glomerulosclerosis. In: Kincaid-Smith P, d'Apice AJF, Atkins R, eds. Progress in Glomerulonephritis. New York, John Wiley and Sons, 1979, 209–228.

8. Habib R, Levy M, Gubler MC: Clinicopathological correlation in the nephrotic syndrome. *Paediatrician* 1979, 8:325.

9. Beaufils H, Alphonse JC, Guedon J, Legain M: Focal global sclerosis: Natural history and treatment. A report of 70 cases. *Nephron.* 1978, 21:75–85.

10. Rydel JJ, Korbet SM, Borok RZ, Schwartz MM. Focal segmental glomerular sclerosis in adults: Presentation, course, and response to treatment. *Am J Kidney Dis.* 1995, 25:534–542.

11. Banfi G, Moriggi M, Sabadini E, Fellin G, D'Amico G, Ponticelli C. The impact of prolonged immunosuppression on the outcome of idiopathic focal-segmental glomerulosclerosis with nephrotic syndrome in adults. A collaborative retrospective study. *Clin Nephrol.* 1991, 36:53–59.

12. Waldher R, Gubler MC, Levy M, Broyer M, Habib R: The significance of pure diffuse mesangial proliferation in idiopathic nephrotic syndrome. *Clini Nephrol.* 1978, 10:171–179.

13. Cameron JS: The natural history of glomerulonephritis. In: Black D, Jones NF, eds. Renal Disease. London: Blackwell Scientific Publishers, 1979, 329–382.

14. Collaborative Study of the Adult Idiopathic Nephrotic Syndrome. A controlled study of short term prednisolone treatment in adults with membranous nephropathy. *New Engl J Med.* 1979, **301**:1301–1306.

15. McEnery PT, McAdams AJ, West CD: Membranoproliferative Glomerulonephritis: improved survival with alternate day prednisolone therapy. *Clin Nephrol.* 1980, **13**:117–124.

16. Kincaid-Smith P: The natural history and treatment of mesangiocapillary glomerulonephritis. In: Kincaid-Smith P, Mathew TH, Becker EC eds. Glomerulonephritis. Morphology, Natural History and Treatment. Part I. New York: John Wiley and Sons, 1973, 591–609.

17. Woo KT: Proteinuria in Renal Disease. Proc 11th Asian Colloquium in Nephrology, Singapore, 1996, 383–391.

18. Woo KT, Lau YK, Yap HK, Lee GSL, Chiang GSC, Lim CH. Protein selectivity: A prognostic index in IgA nephritis. *Nephron.* 1989, **52**:300–306.

19. Remuzzi G, Ruggenenti P, Benigni A. Understanding the nature of renal disease progression. *Kidney Int.* 1997, **51**:2–15.

20. Lewis EJ, Hunsicker LG, Bain RP, Rohde RD for the collaborative study group: The effect of angiotensin coverting enzyme inhibition on Diabetic Nephropathy. *New Engl J Med.* 1993, **329**:456–462.

21. Brenner BM, Meyer TW, Hostetter TH: Dietary protein and the progressive nature of kidney disease. *New Engl J Med.* 1982, **307**:652–659.

22. Woo KT, Lau YK, Lee GSL, Wei SS, Lim CH. Pattern of proteinuria in IgA nephritis by SDS-PAGE: Clinical significance. *Clin Nephrol.* 1991, **36**:6–11.

23. Ponticelli C, Zucchelli P, Passerini P, Cesana B, Locatelli F, Pasquali S et al: A 10 year follow-up of a randomized study with methylprednisolone and chlorambucil in membranous nephropathy. *Kidney Int.* 1995, **48**:1600–1604.

24. MC Cauley J, Shapiro R, Ellis D, Igdal H, T Zakis A, Starzl TE: Pilot trial of FK 506 in the management of steroid resistant

nephrotic syndrome. Nephrology, Dialysis and Transplantation, 1993, **8**:1286–1290.

25. Briggs WA, Choi MJ, Scheel AJ Jr: Successful Mycophenolate Mofetil Treatment of Glomerular Disease. *Am J Kidney Dis.* 1998, **31**:213–217.

CHAPTER 6

Pathogenesis and Therapy of IgA Nephritis

INTRODUCTION

IgA nephritis (IgA Nx) is the commonest form of glomerulonephritis in Singapore accounting for 52% of all primary glomerulonephritis and is therefore a very important cause of end stage kidney failure.[1] Sixty-two percent of patients present with asymptomatic haematuria and proteinuria, 20% with gross or visible haematuria, 8% with the nephrotic syndrome, 7% with chronic renal failure and 3% with acute renal failure associated with crescents on renal biopsy. In IgA Nx there is an immunological defect, likely to be genetic in origin which causes the B lymphocytes of the patient to secrete increased IgA in response to an environmental antigen (microbial or otherwise). The presence of an abnormal T suppressor cell function and augmented T helper cell function results in increased B cells bearing surface IgA and T cells bearing receptors for Fc region of IgA.

Pathogenesis

In the pathogenesis of IgA Nx, four requisites must be present for glomerulonephritis to develop. There must be a propensity for IgA immune complexes (IgAIC) to be deposited in the kidneys. There must be a defective clearance of IgAIC by the kidneys. The mesangial cells of the kidneys must respond by producing certain cytokines capable of eliciting a noxious response which are detrimental to the kidneys. As a result of the noxious response, inflammation or glomerulonephritis occurs, giving rise to haematuria and proteinuria.

Defective Clearance of Immune Complexes

Patients with IgA Nx have defective clearance of IgA coated particles, heat aggregated IgA or IgA-IgG by the liver and spleen.[2] They have a general defect in removal of immune complexes. An individual can have IgAIC within the circulation which is filtered by the kidneys, but as long as the kidneys can get rid of these IgAIC the person will not develop glomerulonephritis. It is only in certain individuals with the disease susceptible gene which makes the kidneys unable to clear these IgAIC that IgA Nx will develop. In addition, IgA binds complements poorly and inhibits complement activation by IgA immune complexes. Complement normally helps to solubulise IC but since the action of complements is inhibited, glomerular deposition of IC is enhanced in IgA Nx.

Role of Cytokines

Recently, cytokines have been found to play an important role in IgA Nx.[3] Interlukin-5 (IL-5) has been shown to selectively increase IgA positive cells which is increased in IgA Nx. IL-6 too is elevated in IgA Nx. Transgenic mice with high IL-6 levels have elevated serum IgA and mesangial proliferative glomerulonephritis (GN) with IgA deposits. IL-6 is mitogenic for mesangial cells. In the presence of IL-6, mesangial cells would undergo proliferation, giving rise to mesangial proliferative glomerulonephritis typical of IgA Nx.

The Propensity for IgA Deposition in IgA Nx

Molecular weight (MW) of IgA, especially polymeric IgA favours deposition in the mesangium because of its larger size. IgA molecules are poorly solubilized by the complement system and allows its deposition in the kidney. IgA is also more anionic than IgG and M and therefore are preferentially deposited in the mesangium which attracts anionic or negatively charged molecules.[3] The mesangial cells bear cationic or positive charges. The IgA eluted from mesangial deposits is also more "anionic" than serum IgA.[4] Urinary albumin in IgA Nx patients too are "anionic".[4] Finally, serum IgA, circulating macromolecular IgA, all have an affinity for the mesangial matrix components like fibronectin and laminin which bear cationic charges.

It is postulated that in patients with IgA Nx there is a defect both in the "sera" (existence of IgAIC) and in the "renal tissue" (abnormal mesangial cells). This would explain the disappearance of IgA Nx from some donated kidneys after transplantation (these kidneys with IgA Nx were inadvertently transplanted), and the recurrence of IgA Nx in those receiving kidneys from living related donors, less so from cadavers.[5] These were patients with IgA Nx as the original disease but the transplanted kidneys did not have IgA Nx at the time of transplantation. In those patients where there is a recurrence of IgA in the kidney without any renal detriment, it would support the theory that lack of genetically mediated mesangial reactivity towards IgA Nx prevents the clinical and histological manifestations of IgA Nx.

Mechanism by which Mesangial Deposits Initiate Glomerular Injury

The binding of IgA deposits to mesangial cells induces certain changes within the mesangial cells causing the secretion of cytokines associated with a decrease in prostaglandin E2 synthesis and increase in thromboxane A2 production promoting mesangial cell proliferation. Elicitation of Angiotensin II also induces mesangial cell contraction and efferent arteriolar vasoconstriction.[6]

IgAIC deposited in the mesangium then bind to mesangial cells and exert their nephritogenic effect through the stimulation of release of cytokines from mesangial cells. Cytokines exert noxious effects causing proliferation of mesangial cells and inflammatory injury which results in glomerulonephritis manifesting as haematuria and proteinuria. Macromolecules which are unable to bind to mesangial cells cannot exert nephritogenicity. The IgA antibody in the IgAIC concentrates and aggregates the antigen into the mesangium, but it is the antigen which is the critical pathogenic component in the equation of nephritogenecity.

Therapeutic Strategies

Various types of food antigen (soya bean protein, gliadin, bovine serum albumin) and infective agents (streptoccous, sendai virus) have been implicated in patients with IgA Nx. It can occur in a sporadic or familial fashion. Currently, it is believed that a disease susceptible gene is involved but no gene has as yet been identified. Some suspect that it is a heterogenous disease with multifactorial etiology.

Any form of therapy must be rational as well as practical. Based on the foregoing discussion on pathogenesis, the ideal therapeutic strategy should attempt to limit the amount of mesangial deposits as well as reduction of noxious glomerular responses to the deposits.[7]

Ways to Limit Amounts of Mesangial Deposits

1. Reduction of antigen load

Gluten-free diet could be recommended for IgA Nx patients who have high levels of IgA directed against gliadin to reduce generation of gliadin/anti-gliadin complexes.[8]

2. Tonsillectomy

This could be considered in patients with chronic tonsillitis because long term follow-up of patients with IgA Nx who have had tonsillectomy have shown that tonsillectomy blunts the progression of IgA Nx.[9]

3. Lymphokines

In view of the significant role played by lymphokines in the pathogenesis of IgA Nx, various forms of therapy could be formulated to downregulate the effects of various lymphokines. The prospect to correct pathogenic immunologic defect induced by lymphokines is challenging. This will be discussed later.

4. Enzymes

Systemically administered enzymes (Dextranase and Protease) have been used to remove glomerular immune deposits in rodents.[10] This has not been tried in patients but the prospects of such a therapy sounds promising.

A Pathophysiologic Approach

The focus for such an approach should be on the mesangial cell responses to immune complexes, complements, cytokines and vasoactive mediators.

1. Immunomodulators

Steroids,[11] Cyclophosphamide[12] and Cyclosporine[13] have been used with varying success in patients with IgA Nx. These agents, since they are immunosuppressants, would attenuate lymphocyte function and serve to downregulate the effects of cytokines in the glomeruli but their toxicity and necessity for continuity limits their applicability. Proteinuria in patients rebounds on stopping the medication.

2. Anti-platelet and anti-thrombotic Therapy

Patients with IgA Nx have evidence of platelet involvement and low grade intravascular coagulation with a tendency for increased thrombogenecity within the kidneys. Use of Dipyridamole (anti-platelet and anti-PDGF agent) and Warfarin (anti-thrombotic agent) have been successful in two separate trials[12,14] in patients with IgA Nx. The relative freedom from side effects and their low cost allow long-term treatment in these patients.

3. ACE inhibitor and Angiotensin II Receptor Antagonist (ATRA)

In IgA Nx, glomerular hyperfiltration injury as evidenced by presence of late onset phase of proteinuria or increasing proteinuria is accompanied by intra-glomerular hypertension due to local hyperactivity of the renin angiotensin system and angiotensin II mediated efferent arteriolar vasoconstriction. The use of ACE or ATRA inhibitor has been shown to be of benefit in reducing proteinuria and preservation of renal function.[15] (See Appendix: Pg 339)

4. Low protein diet

A low protein diet (0.8 gm/kg bw/day) would reduce macromolecular flux and afferent arteriolar vasodilation contributing to glomerular hyperfiltration.

Future Therapeutic Strategies

1. Inhibitors of mediators and cytokines

Drugs like platelet derived growth factor (PDGF) antagonists, tumour necrosis factor (TNF) inhibitor, platelet activating and thromboxane receptor antagonist have not been employed in clinical trials for IgA Nx but they appear to be rational and practical approaches from the pathophysiologic viewpoint. These therapeutic approaches would be directed to inhibit effects of mediators and cytokines involved in IgA Nx.

2. Gene therapy

Gene therapy would offer the ideal therapeutic approach. Modulation of transduction by intracellular signal upon DNA transcription or translation of mRNA may prove effective. One could modulate a specific signal leading to abnormal response to mesangial cells. Another novel approach utilizes "antisense nucleotides". Gene expression in cells is normally regulated by DNA binding proteins, repressors and activators. It was found that complementary nucleic acids could also modulate gene expression. Antisense RNA complementary to regions of mRNA was demonstrated to suppress translation and hence gene expression. Hence, there is a possibility of using synthetic oligonucleotides to regulate gene expression.[16]

In principle, one identifies a unique target sequence in the gene of interest and prepare a complementary oligonucleotide against the target sequence. Antisense DNAs were first utilised against Rous sarcoma virus by Zamecnik and Stephenson in 1978.[17] In IgA Nx, antisense nucleotides could arrest transcription or transduction of a specific mRNA which gives rise to mesangial cell proliferation. Another nucleotide could perhaps switch off the message leading to mesangial cell contraction. It is mesangial cell contraction, following mesangial cell proliferation which leads to mesangial sclerosis, with eventual global glomerulosclerosis and death of that particular glomerulus. It is hoped that therapy in the future may involve antisense nucleotides to modulate abnormal mesangial cell response.

Therapy of IgA Nephritis: Present Status

1. Intraglomerular effect of dipyridamole

Since 1979, Woo et al[12] have used dipyridamole as an anti-platelet agent. Their[18] earlier work on platelet involvement in IgA Nx supported a rationale for its use in combination with low dose warfarin. But relative importance of glomerular platelet infiltration versus direct intraglomerular effect of dipyridamole is not clear. Its anti-platelet effect within the glomerulus may be only one aspect of its effects within the glomerulus.

Recently, dipyridamole has been shown to have an anti-proliferative effect on mesangial cells.[19] It has also been demonstrated to have anti-proliferative effect on smooth muscle endothelial cells.[20] This anti-proliferative effect may be mediated through inhibition of PDGF, a cytokine produced by the mesangial cell and is a potent growth factor for mesangial cells.[21,22] Further work is in progress to determine if dipyridamole also inhibits mesangial cell contractility.

2. Effect of low dose warfarin

Intraglomerular coagulation has been proposed as one of the factors causing glomerular injury in IgA Nx. Yamebe et al[23] demonstrated the presence of Hagmann factor in 68% of 31 patients with IgA Nx using a polyclonal antibody against Factor XII. They postulated that local activation of the contact coagulation factors in the glomeruli initiated intraglomerular coagulation via the intrinsic coagulation systems as well as activating other mediators of inflammation such as kinins and plasmin. In another study by Tan and Woo,[24] plasma concentration of Hagemann factor, pre-kallikrein and high molecular weight kininogen were measured in 24 patients with IgA Nx and 123 normal controls. The plasma titres of all 3 factors measured were significantly lower in IgA Nx compared to controls suggesting activation of the contact coagulation system in IgA Nx.

In IgA Nx, 30% of patients have fibrin deposits within the glomeruli.[25] The above studies by Yamabe,[23] Tan and Woo,[24] and Woo et al's previous documentation of high plasma anti-thrombin III levels in IgA Nx,[26] suggest local intra-vascular coagulation and endothelial cell injury. Warfarin, used in low dose for its anti-thrombotic effect may ameliorate this injury. Lee has also recently demonstrated that warfarin inhibits proliferation of mesangial cells in culture.

Lee and Woo have published the results of a controlled trial using dipyridamole and low dose warfarin in patients with IgA Nx and have shown that such treatment significantly retarded the progression of patients to ESRF.[14] There were 11 patients on treatment and 9 controls, all with renal impairment and serum creatinine ranging from 1.6 mg/dl to 3.0 mg/dl. After 10 months the serum creatinine was higher in the control group but not in the treatment group. At 3 years the findings were similar but 4 from the control group were in end stage renal failure with one in the treatment group. Proteinuria was decreased in the treatment group at 10 months but not in the control group. There was no difference in proteinuria at the end of the trial at 3 years in both groups. This trial has supported the rationale for therapy of patients with IgA Nx and confirmed the findings of an earlier controlled trial by Woo et al.[12]

In an earlier trial,[12] there were 27 patients on treatment and 21 controls. The treatment group was administered cyclophosphamide 1.5 mg/kg bw for 6 months, dipyridamole 300 mg/day and anti-thrombotic dose of warfarin (thrombotest 30% to 50%) for 3 years. In the treatment group, serum creatinine remained unchanged and proteinuria decreased significantly, but in the control group, serum creatinine worsened significantly and proteinuria remained unchanged. Repeat renal biopsies after 3 years showed a worsening in the control group.[27] Both groups were followed up for another

5 years. Those still on treatment with dipyridamole and low dose warfarin (13 patients) had small rises in serum creatinine, but 6 among those who stopped therapy (14 patients) were in end stage renal failure with none in the group still on treatment.[12] It would appear that life long therapy is required to retard progression to end stage renal failure.

Currently, the indications for combination therapy with dipyridamole and low dose warfarin in our Department of Renal Medicine are the presence of any one of the following parameters: proteinuria > 1 gm/day; hypertension; renal impairment; glomerulosclerosis > 20% on renal biopsy; presence of even a single crescent; medial hyperplasia of blood vessels on biopsy.

Our department's guidelines for treatment of patients with IgA Nx with asymptomatic haematuria and proteinuria consist of control of systemic hypertension, use of ACE inhibitor or Angiotensin II Receptor Antagonist (ATRA) for glomerular hyperfiltration, dipyridamole and low dose Warfarin,[32] low protein diet (0.8 gm/Kg BW/day) to reduce macromolecular flux of high protein diet as well as to reduce afferent vasodilation in glomerular hyperfiltration, and control of serum cholesterol to prevent lipid induced glomerulosclerosis.

Diet induced hypercholesterolaemia may be the initiating factor for endothelial cell injury, especially low density lipoprotein (LDL) and very low density lipoprotein (VLDL). Lipoprotein can pass through damaged glomerular filter into the mesangium thereby enhancing the flux of macromolecules and giving rise to hyperperfusion injury.[28] In Japan where IgA nephritis is very common, a similar clinical guideline very close to the one that we are practising has been implemented nationwide in 1995 by a joint committee of the Ministry of Health and Welfare of Japan and the Japanese Society of Nephrology.[29]

For those patients with IgA Nx who have the nephrotic syndrome with selective proteinuria, they should be treated with prednisolone in a dose of 1 mg/kg bw for a month and then gradually tapering and tailing off by the end of 3 months. Those who do not respond to steroids can be given a course of cyclophosphamide at 2 mg/kg bw. The above rationale for therapy is based on our studies on proteinuria involving protein selectivity[30] and iso-electric focussing[31] which showed that although the majority of patients with IgA Nx have diffuse mesangial proliferative glomerulonephritis, as long as they have selective proteinuria they will still respond to steroids.

Those patients who present with acute renal failure associated with more than 20% of crescents on renal biopsy should be offered pulse therapy with methyl prednisolone 0.5 gm daily for 3 successive days or 0.5 gm daily every other day for 6 doses over 12 days. After this, oral prednisolone is prescribed at 1 mg/kg bw with oral cyclophosphamide 2 mg/kg bw. Prednisolone dosage should be reduced gradually over 6 months and stopped and cyclophosphamide maintained at the same dose for 6 months and then stopped. Patients should be on long term maintenance therapy with dipyridamole and anti-thrombotic doses of warfarin. Patients with rapidly progressive glomerulonephritis (more than 50% crescents on renal biopsy) should in addition have plasmapheresis during the first 3 to 4 weeks of therapy.

About 13% of our patients with IgA Nx have predominant tubular interstitial lesions out of proportion to the degree of glomerular sclerosis. These patients should be treated with a low dose of steroid regimen, 30 mg/day of prednisolone for two months, with gradual dose reduction to 10 mg/day by six months and then long term maintenance of 5 to 10 mg/day. This is to retard ischemic renal damage induced by fibrosis of the post capillary vessel of the glomerulus due to fibrosis of the adjacent tubulo-interstitium.

CONCLUSION

IgA nephritis as a vasculitides has similarities to diabetic nephropathy in that both diseases have mesangial proliferation and sclerosis and glomerular hyperfiltration injury which contribute to progressive disease. The current treatment protocol and strategies for both diseases are therefore very similar. Whilst there is no cure for both these types of kidney disease, such therapeutic measures serve to retard the progression to end stage renal failure. Future therapeutic strategies lie in immunomodulation using inhibitors of cytokines and possibly gene therapy.

REFERENCES

1. Woo KT, Edmondson RPS, Wu AYT, Chiang GSC, Pwee HS, Lim CH. The natural history of IgA nephritis in Singapore. *Clin Nephrol.* 1986, **25**:15–21.

2. Rocatello D, Picciotto G, Coppo R, Piccoli G, Molino A, Cacace G et al. Clearance of polymeric IgA aggregates in humans. *Am J Kidney Disease.* 1989, **14**:354–360.

3. Gallo GR, Caulin-Glaser T, Emancipator SN, Lamm SE. Nephritogenecity and differential distribution of glomerular immune complexes are related to immunogen charge. *Lab Invest.* 1983, **48**:353–361.

4. Woo KT, Lau YK, Lee GSL, Wong KS, Chin YM, Chiang GSC, Lim CH. Isoelectric focussing and protein selectivity index as predictors of response to therapy in IgA nephrotic syndrome. *Nephron.* 1994, **67**:408–413.

5. Brensilver JN, Mallat S, Scholes J, Mc Cabe R. Recurrent IgA nephropathy in living related donor transplantation: Recurrence or transmission of familial disease? *Am J Kidney Dis.* 1988, **2**:147–151.

6. Rifai A, Chen A, Imai H. Complement activation in experimental IgA nephropathy: An antigen mediated process. *Kidney Int.* 1987, **32**:838–844.

7. Clarkson AR, Woodroffe AJ, Aarons IA, Thompson T, Hale GM. Therapeutic options in IgA nephropathy. *Am J Kidney Dis.* 1988, **12**:443–448.

8. Coppo R, Rocatello D, Amore A, Quattrocchio G, Molino A, Gianoglio B. et al. Effects of gluten-free diet in primary IgA nephropathy. *Clin Nephrol.* 1990, **33**:72–86.

9. Bene MC, De Ligny GH, Kessler M, Faure G. Confirmation by tonsillar anomalies in IgA nephropathy: A multicenter study. *Nephron.* 1991, **58**:425–428.

10. Gesualdo L, Ricanati S, Hassan MO, Emancipator SN, Lamm ME. Enzymolysis of glomerular immune deposits in vivo with dextranase/protease ameliorates proteinuria, hematuria and mesangial proliferation in murine experimental IgA nephropathy. *J Clin Invest.* 1990, **86**:715–722.

11. Kobayashi Y, Yoshiyuki H, Kazufumi F, Kurokawa A, Tateno S. IgA nephropathy: Heterogenous clinical picture and steroid therapy in progressive cases. *Semin Nephrol.* 1987, **7**:382–385.

12. Woo KT, Lee GSL, Lau YK, Chiang GSC, Lim CH. Effects of triple therapy in IgA nephritis: A follow up study 5 years later. *Clin Nephrol.* 1991, **36**:60–66.

13. Lai KN, Lai FM. Short term controlled trial of cyclosporine A in IgA nephritis. Abstract, Second International Symposium on IgA Nephritis, Bari, Italy. 1987, pg 34.

14. Lee GSL, Woo KT, Lim CH. Controlled trial of dipyridamole and low dose warfarin in patients with IgA nephritis with renal impairment. *Clin Nephrol.* 1989, **31**:276.

15. Woo KT, Lau YK, Wong KS, Chiang GSC. ACE/ATRA therapy decrease proteinuria by improving glomerular permselectivity in IgA nephritis. *Kidney Int.* 2000, **58**:2485–2491.

16. Agrawal G. Antisense oligonucleotides: *A possible approach for chemotherapy of AIDS*. In: Eric Wichstrom, editor. Prospects for Antisense Nucleic Acid Therapy of Cancer and AIDS. New York, USA: Wiler-Liss, 1991:143–158.

17. Zamecnik PC, Stephenson ML. Inhibition of rous-sarcoma virus replication and cell transformation by a specific oligodeoxyribonucleotide. *Proc Nat Acad Sci*, USA. 1978, **75**:280–284.

18. Woo KT, Tan YO, Yap HK, Lau YK, Lim CH. Beta-thromboglobulin in mesangial IgA nephritis. *Thromb Res.* 1981, **24**:259–262.

19. Lee GSL, Woo KT, Tan HB, Lim CH. Effects of Dipyridamole in Mesangial Cell Proliferation and Collagen Synthesis in Cultures of Rat Mesangial Cells. *28th Singapore-Malaysian Congress of Medicine*, 1994, Abstract, pg 67(b).

20. Choong HL, Tan HB, Woo KT. Proliferation of vascular smooth muscle cells is attenuated by dipyridamole. *28th Singapore-Malaysian Congress of Medicine*, 1994, Abstract, pg 67(a).

21. Silver BJ, Jaffer FE, Abboud HE. Platelet derived growth factor synthesis in mesangial cells: Induction by multiple peptide mitogens. *Proc Natl Acad Sci*, USA. 1989, **86**:1056.

22. Abboud HE: Resident glomerular cells in glomerular injury: Mesangial cells. *Semin Nephrol.* 1991, **11**:304–310.

23. Yamabe H, Sugawara N, Ozawa K, Kubota H, Fukushi K, Kikuchi K, Onodera K. Glomerular deposition of Hagmann Factor in IgA nephritis. *Nephron.* 1984, **37**:62–63.

24. Tan CC, Woo KT. Plasma contact coagulation factors in IgA nephritis. *Ann Acad Med*, S'pore, 1996, **25**:218–221.

25. Woo KT, Chiang GSC, Lau YK, Lim CH. IgA nephritis in Singapore: Clinical, prognostic indices and therapy. *Semin Nephrol.* 1987, **7**:379–381.

26. Woo KT, Lee EJC, Lau YK, Lim CH. Anti-thrombin III in mesangial IgA nephritis. *Thromb Res.* 1985, **40**:483–487.

27. Woo KT, GSC Chiang, Lim CH. Follow up renal biopsies in IgA nephritic patients on triple therapy. *Clin Nephrol.* 1987, **28**:304–305.

28. Diamond JR, Karnovsky MJ. Focal and segmental glomerulosclerosis: Analogies to atherosclerosis. *Kidney Int.* 1988, **33**:917–924.

29. Sakai H, Abe K, Kobayashi Y, Koyama A, Shigematsu H, Harada T et al. Clinical guidelines of IgA nephropathy. *Japanese J of Nephrol.* 1995, **37**:417–421.

30. Woo KT, Lau YK, Yap HK, Lee GSL, Chiang GSC, Lim CH. Protein selectivity: A prognostic index in IgA nephritis. *Nephron.* 1989, **52**:300–306.

31. Woo KT, Lau YK, Wong KS, Lee GSL, Chin YM, Chiang GSC, Lim CH. Isoelectric focussing and selectivity index in IgA nephrotic syndrome. *Nephron.* 1994, **67**:408–413.

32. Woo KT, Lee GSL, Pall AA. Dipyridamole and low dose warfarin without cyclophosphamide in the management of IgA nephropathy. *Kidney Int.* 2000, **57**:348–349.

CHAPTER 7

Lupus Nephritis

Renal Involvement in Systemic Lupus Erythematosus (SLE)

Fifty to ninety per cent of patients with SLE have nephritis. It affects the glomeruli, tubules and blood vessels of the kidneys. The onset can be insidious to precipitous. This is a chronic disease with remissions and exacerbations. Women are more likely to be affected by SLE.

Assessment of the Patient at Presentation

1. In the clinical assessment of the patient, one has to determine whether the patient has asymptomatic lupus nephritis (urinary abnormalities) or features of the nephrotic syndrome.
2. The younger age group and male patients do worse.
3. Determine whether the patient has hypertension.
4. If there is renal failure, determine whether it is acute, chronic or acute on chronic renal failure. Acute renal failure is potentially reversible. Acute renal deterioration in a patient with lupus nephritis could be due to sepsis, transformation of the lupus nephritis to one with a more severe histology, a crescenteric change (rapidly progressive glomerulonephritis), pre-renal failure due to the nephrotic syndrome, uncontrolled hypertension, renal vein thrombosis, drugs like non-steroidal anti-inflammatory drugs (NSAIDS) or nephrotoxic antibiotics.

Investigations

1. Urine examination: A telescoped specimen (presence of RBC, WBC, casts and protein) points to the likelihood of diffuse lupus nephritis. Culture the urine if infection is suspected.
2. Full blood counts, platelets. If there is anaemia, proceed to a reticulocyte count, Coomb's test, peripheral blood film.
3. Serum creatinine, creatinine clearance.
4. Total urinary protein in 24 hours' urine collection.
5. Total serum protein, serum albumin.
6. Anti-nuclear factor, anti-DNA, serum complement.
7. Chest X-ray if chest infection suspected.
8. Ultrasound of the kidneys and renal biopsy.

Renal Biopsy

Some advocate a renal biopsy for all patients because of "silent nephritis", ie. no urinary abnormalities but a renal biopsy shows lupus nephritis.

Others perform a biopsy only if urinary abnormalities are present. A renal biopsy is useful as it will help to determine the type and extent of the renal pathology. It helps in the planning of the management as well as the rendering of a prognosis. A biopsy also helps in the interpretation of the renal failure as to whether the renal failure is reversible (acute renal failure) or chronic.

WHO Classification of Lupus Nephritis

Class I. Normal glomeruli
— Nil change
— Normal LM, deposits by IMF or EM

Class II.   Pure mesangial alterations

Class III.   Focal segmental glomerulonephritis
Associated with mild or moderate mesangial alterations. May be proliferative, necrotising or sclerosing (< 50% glomeruli involved). Necrosis and leukocytic infiltration indicate a higher degree of activity. More aggressive clinical course than Class II. Class III and IV are continuation of the same lesion.

Class IV.   Diffuse glomerulonephritis
— Associated with severe mesangial, endocapillary or mesangio-capillary proliferation and/or extensive subendothelial deposits.
— Majority of glomeruli involved with hypercellularity. There are focal areas of necrosis, crescents, nuclear debris and wire loops.
— IMF may show full house immunoglobulins and EM will show subendothelial deposits.
— Patients usually have a severe clinical picture with nephrotic range proteinuria and active urinary sediment, and renal impairment occurs more frequently.

Class V.   Diffuse membranous glomerulonephritis
This lesion has a better prognosis than Class III and IV.

Class VI.   Advanced sclerosing glomerulonephritis
The prognosis is not good as many will develop renal failure.

Indices of Activity and Chronicity

These indices or lesions (see below) represent active (potentially reversible) lesions → Activity Index, or chronic, sclerosing, fibrosing (presumably irreversible) lesions → Chronicity Index. A graded scale consists of 0, 1, 2, and 3+. The total score forms an INDEX; Activity or Chronicity Index as the case may be.

Active Lesions (Potentially Reversible)

1. Disruption of capillary walls
2. Polymorphs and karyorrhexis
3. Haematoxyphil bodies
4. Crescents
5. Wire loops
6. Hyaline thrombi
7. Fibrin thrombi
8. Segmental fibrin deposition

Activity index is a relatively weak predictor of renal failure outcome. Mild to moderate elevations of the index represent reversible disease (with treatment). A marked elevation of index may represent disruption of glomerular capillaries which tend to heal by scarring rather than regression. Cellular crescents and severe fibrinoid necrosis are the most ominous. The presence of subendothelial deposit is evidence of activity and is an indicator for treatment.

Chronic Lesions (Irreversible)

1. Segmental sclerosis
2. Mesangial sclerosis

3. Global sclerosis
4. Fibrous crescents
5. Interstitial fibrosis
6. Tubular atrophy

Chronicity index has a graded relationship to risk of ESRF as a high index appears to increase the risk of renal functional deterioration.

Renal Histopathology and Survival (Baldwin 1977)

1. Focal glomerulonephritis
   — 92% normal renal function
   — 2/3 of patients are nephrotic
   — 70% five-year survival

2. Membranous glomerulonephritis
   — proteinuria present in nearly all patients — 70% of patients are nephrotic
   — 79% five-year survival

3. Diffuse proliferative glomerulonephritis
   — 90% of patients have nephrotic syndrome
   — 82% have renal impairment
   — 30% five-year survival

Serologic Parameters (Balow)

1. Serum complement (CH50, C3, C4) usually correlates with degree of activity of glomerular disease.
2. Falling levels of complement predict lupus flare.
3. Immunosuppressive drugs usually improve C3 levels and this would correlate with reduction of disease activity.

4. Others: anti-DNA antibodies, circulating immune complexes, and C reactive protein are useful but none of the tests "alone" are specific or sensitive enough as strict guides to therapy, activity or prognosis.

Correlation between Serologic Markers and Disease Activity (Hayslett)

1. High titres of anti-DNA and haemolytic complement (CH50) is associated with active disease and their absence indicates inactivity.
2. An increase in anti-DNA or fall in CH50 heralds relapse by several weeks.
3. The solid phase C1q binding assay for circulating immune complexes also correlates with activity.
4. Normalisation of anti-DNA and CH50 with treatment is associated with a better outcome.

Assessment of a Patient for Therapy

When assessing a patient for therapy one has to consider:

1. Whether the patient has nephrotic syndrome, hypertension or renal impairment.
2. Determine if active disease is present.
3. A renal biopsy will help to determine the type of lesion, the activity index and the chronicity index.

Assessment for Pregnancy

1. Does patient have active disease? Check urinary sediment and lupus markers.
2. What is the renal function like?

3. Does she have hypertension?
4. Is there proteinuria and if so, is it heavy?
5. Are complement levels and anti-DNA titres low or normal?
6. A renal biopsy will enable one to assess the activity and chronicity indices.

Pregnancy In Women with SLE

1. Pregnancy increases exacerbations of SLE. These exacerbations are higher during pregnancy and in the post-partum period.
2. Patients with complete remission a few months prior to conception have lower incidence of relapses (25% to 35%).
3. Those with active disease in pregnancy have 50% to 60% incidence of exacerbations.
4. There is a 90% foetal survival for those with inactive SLE and 50% to 75% for those with active SLE.
5. The presence of lupus anticoagulant causes thrombosis in the placenta resulting in intrauterine deaths and abortions.

Treatment of Lupus Nephritis

1. High dose prednisolone (45 mg or 60 mg) for 3 months, then reduce to 20 mg over 3 months for those with nephrotic syndrome and those who have mild to moderate Class IV nephritis. Maintain with 10 mg a day.
2. Prednisolone and oral cyclophosphamide (2 mg/kg body weight) for 6 months, then prednisolone alone for non-steroid responsive nephrotic syndrome and those with moderate Class IV nephritis. Those who fail Cyclophosphamide can be offered CyA at 5 mg/kg BW for 3 months with dose reduction over the next 3 months.
3. Prednisolone and oral cyclophosphamide for 12 months, then prednisolone alone for moderate to severe Class IV

(those who have crescents, fibrin thrombi and sclerosis on renal biopsy). Patients with diffuse sclerosing lesions or renal impairment should also be offered the same treatment. If fail, try Cyclosporine A and maintain up to 1 year.

4. Pulse methyprednisolone (0.5 gm I.V. daily for 6 days) with oral cyclophosphamide and prednisolone for a year for those with acute renal deterioration where biopsies show active Class IV with crescents and fibrin thrombi (High activity index).

5. Oral cyclophosphamide with maintenance prednisolone or Azathioprine with prednisolone for those with biopsies showing sclerosis and fibrous crescents with mild renal impairment (High chronicity index).

6. Plasmapheresis for those with rapidly progressive glomerulonephritis or pulmonary haemorrhage.

7. Patients with Class II (pure mesangial) or Class V (membranous) lupus nephritis should have only low dose steroid therapy unless they are nephrotic, in which case remission could be induced with high dose prednisolone. Cyclophosphamide or Azathioprine for 6 months could be used if there is no response to prednisolone.

8. Patients with Class VI (diffuse sclerosing) lesions with serum creatinine above 450 micro Mol/L or 5 mg/dl should not be treated aggressively. They require protein restriction, control of hypertension and treatment for sepsis, as well as plans for long-term renal replacement therapy.

Increased Risk of Mortality

The following are features associated with an increased risk of ESRF:

1. Severe proteinuria during early clinical course
2. Renal impairment

3. Diffuse proliferative lupus nephritis (Class IV)
4. High chronicity index (sclerosis, crescents, interstitial fibrosis and tubular atrophy)
5. Younger age at disease onset
6. Male gender

Predictors of Mortality

The following are predictors of mortality in any patient with SLE:

1. Severe proteinuria during early clinical course
2. Renal impairment
3. Anaemia from any cause
4. Central nervous system disease (any form)
5. Younger age at disease onset
6. Disease duration prior to SLE diagnosis

Prognosis

1. The overall 10-year survival rate is 70%.
2. The risk of ESRF within 10 years is 30% for those with diffuse proliferative lupus nephritis.
3. Young age and male gender increase the risk of renal failure.
4. Patients with insidious progression of azotaemia are likely to develop chronic irreversible disease.
5. A swift decline in renal function means active, treatable and potentially reversible lupus nephritis.

CHAPTER 8

Urinary Tract Infection

The diagnosis of urinary tract infection is based on the demonstration of bacteria in the urine. Urine specimens can be obtained in one of 3 ways.

1. Mid Stream Urine

The patient should start with a full bladder, preferably the morning specimen. In the case of a female patient, a tampon should be used to prevent vaginal secretions from contaminating the urine specimen. The labia should be separated. In the uncircumcised male, the foreskin should be retracted. The exposed surface should then be cleansed with normal saline. After this the patient voids the first 200 ml of urine. Without stopping the micturition stream, the container is passed under the stream and the urine collected. The mid stream specimen of urine is then sent for urine microscopy as well as for culture and sensitivity. If colony counts exceed 10^5 it denotes an infection.

2. Suprapubic Aspiration

This is the best method for determining significant bacteriuria. Any bacterial growth regardless of the numbers is significant.

3. Catheterised Specimen

If for any reason the mid stream urine cannot be obtained or a suprapubic aspiration is contraindicated, then one may have to resort to a catheterised urine specimen. This method of obtaining urine should be the last resort as it carries the danger of introducing urinary tract infection. Remember to instill 100 ml of 0.2% neomycin in the bladder before removing the catheter.

EVIDENCE OF URINARY TRACT INFECTION

Direct evidence of urinary infection is provided by demonstration of bacterial growth in the urine.

Indirect evidence is provided by the demonstration of pyuria exceeding 3 WBC per high power field. For the modified Addis count where the cell count in 1 ml of urine is determined, the following are abnormal: WBC > 2000/ml, RBC > 800/ml and casts > 1000/ml.

The mid stream urine should be cultured within 30 minutes. If at night, the urine specimen should be refrigerated if it cannot be sent off to the laboratory. Sometimes one can have a colony count of less than 10^5 which could still represent an infection, eg. if the patient has symptoms in the afternoon and he drinks a lot of fluid, the counts may be low. A mixed growth in general means a contaminated specimen. If 3 organisms are isolated together there is only a 5% incidence of this being due to an infection.

STERILE PYURIA

In a patient with sterile pyuria one has to exclude anaerobes, bacteriophage and mycoplasma. For the isolation of such organisms one requires a special culture medium. Fungal infection is another cause of sterile pyuria. A patient who has earlier received antibiotics from his general practitioner before coming to see you may not grow any organisms from his urine as the antibiotic is still present in his urine. Sometimes bacteriuria may be intermittent. Tuberculosis is of course a well-known cause of sterile pyuria and one should always remember to send urine for AFB cultures. In a woman, cancer of the cervix is something to remember and a vaginal examination may be indicated. Reflux nephropathy, analgesic nephropathy and renal stones are other causes of sterile pyuria.

SYMPTOMS

The symptoms of urinary infection in an adult are frequency of micturition, dysuria, bladder discomfort, loin pain, and fever with rigors. The presence of gross haematuria usually means involvement of the bladder indicating the presence of cystitis. This in a woman may be a clue to sexually related bladder infection or honeymoon cystitis.

In a patient with acute symptomatic urinary tract infection, about 25% of cultures will be sterile or there will be no significant counts. Of the other 75%, colony counts will exceed 10^5, half of whom would have cystitis and the other half an upper tract infection (pyelonephritis).

RADIOLOGY

An intravenous pyelogram is traditionally indicated in a male even if it is a first infection. In the case of a female the IVP is indicated only on the second infection. This is because females with a shorter urethra are more easily prone to develop cystitis during the sexual act as the urethra is very close to the anus and organisms are often accidentally introduced during sexual intercourse.

The IVP may show chronic atrophic pyelonephritis through the presence of unilateral or bilateral asymmetrical scars associated with distortion of the pelvicalyceal system. The scars are most often present in the upper poles of the kidneys, then the lower poles, followed by the mid zone. Sometimes an IVP may show renal stones, papillary necrosis or polycystic kidneys.

A Woman with Recurrent Infection

In a woman of child bearing age or for that matter, any female capable of the sexual act, if she has lower tract symptoms (cystitis) and the IVP is normal, the infection is often related to sexual intercourse. In such a case the patient should be given advice on sexual hygiene. Within 15 minutes of sexual intercourse she should empty her bladder. The couple may have to prolong the period of foreplay to ensure that there is adequate lubrication, otherwise they may have to resort to the use of lubricant in the form of KY jelly or other lubricant gel.

If the patient returns with a history of recurrent cystitis in spite of the above measures, then one would have to prescribe a tablet of nitrofurantoin postcoitally. If she returns again with infection the next step is to prescribe a tablet of nitrofurantoin every night. If the infection recurs, then she would require a tablet in the morning and another in the night. Nalidixic acid can also be used as a prophylactic agent though nitrofurantoin is preferable as there is less likelihood of the organism developing resistance. However, nitrofurantoin sometimes gives rise to the unpleasant side effects of nausea and vomiting in individuals who are susceptible. Half a tablet of Bactrium can also be used for prophylaxis.

A Man with Recurrent Infection

In a man with recurrent urinary infection in the presence of a normal IVP, one has to suspect prostatitis and proceed to do a prostatic massage. In the choice of antibiotics remember to choose those that cross into the prostatic bed, namely, ciprofloxacin, erythromycin, trimethoprim, and oleandomycin. In the treatment of prostatic infection one has to continue for a period of 6 weeks to even 3 months.

TREATMENT

For the acute infection there is no difference whether one treats the patient for 6 weeks, 2 weeks or even 1 week. If the patient responds to the antibiotic, the urine should be sterile within a few hours. Symptoms may persist for another 24 to 48 hours. Pyuria however takes about a week to disappear.

One should start off with the simple antibiotics like nitrofurantoin, nalidixic acid or amoxycillin. If symptoms are severe one may want to start with bactrium or ciprofloxacin. A mid stream urine is taken before the commencement of antibiotics and if there is no response, the subsequent choice of antibiotics is dictated by the results of culture and sensitivity. It may be that one may have to prescribe more potent antibiotics like an aminoglycoside such as gentamicin or amikacin or use a cephalosporin. When using an aminoglycoside one should always check the serum creatinine as the dose may have to be reduced in the presence of renal impairment. It is imperative that the levels of gentamicin or amikacin be monitored in the presence of renal impairment so as to prevent nephrotoxicity.

If culture and sensitivity results are not known and the patient is very ill or septicaemic, one should proceed to a combination of an aminoglycoside and amoxycillin intravenously or a cephalosporin. Oral antibiotics like ciprofloxacin 250 mg BD or Zinnat (cefuroxime axetil) 250 mg BD may also be used in a severe infection, provided the patient is not septicaemic.

Single Dose Therapy

Another mode of treatment is Single Dose Therapy. This treatment should be confined to patients who present with symptoms of cystitis. The treatment consists of a single intramuscular injection of 0.5 gm of kanamycin. A single oral dose of Ciprofloxacin 500 mg, Amoxycillin 3 gm or bactrium (4 tablets) may also be used. In Asian women however, big dosage of bactrium may cause headaches with nausea and vomiting.

If there is no response to Single Dose Therapy when the patient returns after a week the patient should have an IVP to exclude any anatomical abnormality. By this time results of cultures and sensitivity would also be ready if it had been sent off earlier.

CONDITIONS ASSOCIATED WITH PYELONEPHRITIS

Conditions associated with pyelonephritis are obstruction to the urinary system, developmental causes like congenital valves, cystic disease and vesicoureteric reflux. Other causes are pregnancy, diabetes mellitus, stones, gout and analgesic abuse. The above list should be thought of in patients with recurrent infections.

Vesicoureteric Reflux

In man, the vesicoureteric valve is extremely competent due to the long intramural segment. Under certain conditions, reflux is demonstrated, eg. during cystitis when the inflamed mucosal valve flap and the intramural ureter is rendered a rigid plastic tube. The refluxing valve is often due to a congenital weakness and the natural history of vesicoureteric reflux is one of spontaneous cure as the valve matures with the growth of the patient.

There are other causes of vesicoureteric reflux apart from a congenital defect. These could be acquired ureteric, bladder or urethral defects, bladder neck obstruction, diverticulum, ureterocele, ectopic ureter, duplex kidneys and renal stones.

In the West, vesicoureteric reflux accounts for 30% of renal failure in children and 15 to 20% in adults (about 10% in Singapore). The radiological term of chronic pyelonephritis which refers to the presence of asymmetrical scars in the kidneys associated with distortion of the pelvicalyceal system should in practice refer to chronic atrophic pyelonephritis which is due to vesicoureteric reflux. In other words acute pyelonephritis should not give rise to renal scars. It is only chronic atrophic pyelonephritis caused by vesicoureteric reflux which causes renal scarring.

Reflux nephropathy or chronic atrophic pyelonephritis affects 1 in 300 of the White female population. Of the number affected, about 10% have a bad prognosis. We do not have any local figures but it is suspected that the incidence is much lower here. However, there is a possibility that the condition may be under diagnosed as micturating cystourethrograms are not performed as frequently. In the West, apart from being an important cause of renal failure it is also a cause of renal hypertension. It has also been found to cause glomerulonephritis where the patients have proteinuria, sometimes in the nephrotic range, and the glomerular lesions are those of focal and segmental glomerulosclerosis. The cause of these glomerular lesions could be due to hyperfiltration, atypical bacterial forms, Tamm Horsfall proteins or an autoimmune basis.

The most important aspect of reflux nephropathy is that it is an important cause of persistent and recurrent urinary infection which can sometimes be very debilitating to the patient plus the fact that it is a cause of chronic renal failure.

The Scarring Process in Man

It has now been shown that in order to form renal scars, 3 conditions must be present. The patient must have composite (compound) renal papillae which allow intrarenal reflux. On this background there must be reflux of infected urine before renal scars can be formed.

Once scars are formed they will progress inexorably and lead to eventual contraction or fibrosis. A 3 cm scar may with time become only a 2 mm fibrous tissue. The patterns of the scars could be confined to the upper poles, bipolar, bilateral focal but unequal, or generalised.

Fresh scars are uncommon after the age of 5 years. The prognosis is poorer if there is no compensatory hypertrophy and the kidneys are progressively getting smaller. In other words, if the patient's infection is suppressed or prevented with prophylactic antibiotics and the reflux has disappeared as the vesicoureteric valves mature, the kidney may grow.

Treatment

As part of the management, a micturating cystourethrogram should be performed and the reflux graded. Grade I is when there is reflux up to the pelvic brim. Grade II is reflux up to the renal pelvis but without causing distension of the pelvis. Grade III is when there is distension of the renal pelvis. Grade IV is when there is intrarenal reflux. However, there can be variability of grading from time to time as bacterial toxins during an infection may cause ureteric dilatation and increase the grading severity.

Children should be on prophylactic antibiotics till after the age of 5 years. After that if they still get infection they should be on prophylactic antibiotics until they are free of infection for 3 years in a stretch. The same applies to adults, especially in the presence of Grade III or IV reflux.

There is no place for routine ureteric reimplantation. The only indication is when the patient has Grade IV reflux in the presence of severe uncontrolled infection and progressive scarring. Another indication is the adult who has pain in the kidney during micturition due to distension of the renal pelvis resulting from urine refluxing during micturition.

Controlled trials have shown that the results of surgery for reimplantation of the ureters are no better than in patients treated medically with prophylactic antibiotics. Besides, the natural history of vesicoureteric reflux is one of spontaneous cure as the vesicoureteric valves mature.

Patients with vesicoureteric reflux with reflux nephropathy, especially if they already have renal impairment may do poorly during pregnancy and may deteriorate to end stage renal failure as a result of pregnancy. It may be safer to advise termination of pregnancy therefore in the presence of renal impairment especially if the patient is also hypertensive.

MANAGEMENT OF RECURRENT URINARY TRACT INFECTION

In the management of a patient with urinary tract infection (UTI), the clinician should take note of two salient features. The first is that clinical improvement does not equate with bacteriologic eradication and the second, follow-up urine cultures are necessary to ensure a cure. The first will determine the choice of antibiotics and the duration of treatment, and the second will help the clinician decide when to do follow-up urine cultures and sensitivity.

Relapsing Recurrences due to Urologic Abnormalities

One should always consider three common causes: renal stone disease, vesicoureteric reflux and prostatitis. A relapse often occurs about two weeks after an infection. In a female, she should receive another 6-week course of treatment and in a male, another 12 weeks. These 6 weeks would ensure proper eradication of UTI due to vesicoureteric reflux and 12 weeks for chronic prostatitis.[1] Relapse occurs because the bacteria are deep-seated within the stone, the prostate or within the kidney tissue in the case of reflux nephropathy. A short course of antibiotic will kill the organism but those within the stone or organ will still survive and cause a relapse if not properly eradicated.

Reinfections

Patients with frequent reinfections will have altered bacteria flora, reflecting faecal bacterial reservoir and impact of antibiotics. Sulphonamides, penicillin and cephalosporins will eradicate gram negative organisms in the gastrointestinal tract

(GIT) but they are replaced by enterobacteraceae or pseudomonas species. The next "infection" usually occurs within 2 to 4 weeks and would be resistant to the above antibiotics. The choice of antibiotics would depend on the results of culture and sensitivity. Nitrofurantoin, trimethoprim and quinolones (nalidixic acid, ciprofloxacin) less commonly select resistant organisms in the GIT.[2]

Prophylaxis

Prophylaxis of symptomatic lower tract infection in women is effective. Women with 2 or more symptomatic upper tract infections in a year should have prophylaxis. Nitrofurantoin 50 mg, cotrimoxazole 240 mg or $\frac{1}{2}$ tablet, nalidixic acid 500 mg following sexual intercourse is effective. If the patient continues to have recurrent infection the antibiotic can be prescribed thrice weekly or even nightly if necessary. In males, there are no definitive studies regarding the value of preventing asymptomatic infection to reduce occurrence of acute pyelonephritis. For patients with vesicoureteric reflux, prophylaxis prevents infection of kidneys, protects or preserves renal function and in a growing child, allows resumption of normal renal growth.[3]

Continuous Suppression

Permanent suppression is recommended in patients with frequent relapses (3 or more episodes a year) or for those where the source of infection cannot be removed, like stones, vesicoureteric reflux, prostatitis or obstructive uropathy.

The suppressive regimen consists of nightly, twice daily or full dose suppressive therapy with nitrofurantoin, cotrimoxazole or nalidixic acid. For example, a patient with chronic prostatitis, after treatment of the infection for 6 to 12 weeks with antibiotics can be put on cotrimoxazole one tablet (480 mg) nightly for years with no infection. It is important to review the patient every 3 to 4 months with urine culture and sensitivity. In the event of a breakthrough infection occurring, a new antibiotic is prescribed to treat the infection. After that, the patient is put on suppressive antibiotics again. Cotrimoxazole can still be used as the suppressive agent once the infection is eradicated. After 2 years on suppressive therapy, in the absence of infection, the antibiotic can be stopped to see if infection recurs. If it does, the patient will require treatment followed by further suppressive therapy.

Patient with Renal Impairment

Aminoglycosides like gentamicin and amikacin should be avoided if possible. If they have to be used, the dose should be reduced and serum creatinine and antibiotic levels monitored. Nitrofurantoin is contraindicated because it is of no use since it is poorly concentrated in the failing kidney. But more importantly, it causes very severe and painful peripheral neuropathy in patients with renal impairment.[4]

Penicillins can be used. The newer ones with a broader spectrum of activity like piperacillin, mezlocillin and azlocillin are also active against most strains or pseudomonas and strep faecalis.[5] They are preferred over the third generation cephalosporins like ceftriazone and ceftazidime if either of these are infecting pathogens. The first generation cephalosporins are nephrotoxic but the second generation is less so and the third generation are safe but dosage has to be reduced in renal failure. Cotrimoxazole consists of trimethoprim which is not nephrotoxic but sulphamethoxazole is. In mild renal impairment only half the usual dose of cotrimoxazole (480 mg) twice daily should be used. Quinolones are safe drugs to use in renal failure.

Causes of recurrent UTI

Recurrent UTI could be due to or associated with the following: obstruction of the urinary tract, vesicoureteric reflux, renal calculi, diabetes mellitus, analgesic nephropathy, polycystic kidneys, cystitis, prostatitis, pregnancy, neurogenic bladder, urinary catheterisation, benign prostatic hypertrophy and uterovaginal prolapse among the elderly.

Obstruction of the Urinary Tract

Obstruction at all levels, from renal tubules to urethral meatus, is the most important factor predisposing to infection. Stasis compromises bladder and renal defence to Sepsis. In patients with renal cortical scars as in reflux nephropathy, there is no increased susceptibility to infection. However in those with renal papillary scars (analgesic nephropathy, diabetic papillary necrosis) there is an increased susceptibility to infection because of intratubular obstruction.

Causes of obstruction could be due to congenital lesions (valves, bands, stenosis, bladder neck obstruction), extrinsic compression of the ureters (tumours, retroperitoneal fibrosis), localised intrarenal obstruction to urinary flow (nephrocalcinosis, uric acid nephropathy, polycystic kidney and analgesic nephropathy).

Vesicoureteric Reflux (VUR)

This is a common cause of UTI. In patients with VUR, bladder infection may induce reflux because the inflamed intramural portion of the ureter is rendered a rigid plastic tube by the inflammation thus allowing reflux when the bladder contracts during micturition. Reflux disappears once infection is controlled. This is therefore a vicious cycle. Infection produces reflux or aggravates it, which in turn maintains the infection by producing residual urine which predisposes to infection because of urinary stasis.

If urinary infection is controlled, reflux tends to diminish as a result of the ureteral and bladder wall growing thicker with age. Prophylactic antibiotics are useful in preventing infection. About 20% of children not on prophylaxis develop new scars compared to those on prophylaxis.[6-8]

Infection and Nephrolithiasis

Damage to renal papillae produced by infection can cause calcified foci which with time become renal stones. The renal stones then cause UTI, incidence varying from 2% to as high as 47%.[9] About 50% of infections are due to proteus mirabilis. UTI with urea splitting organism causes triple phosphate (struvite) stones. There is a 25% mortality over 5 years in patients with stones induced by bilateral renal infection. The risk of stone recurrence after surgery is 40% to 60%. The rate of persistent UTI is 40% because bacteria survive deep inside the stone.[10] In the management of such patients it is important to continue suppressive antibiotic therapy to prevent infected stones.

Diabetes Mellitus

Diabetes mellitus is said to be associated with an increased frequency of UTI. However, this is based on evidence from uncontrolled or poorly controlled studies. A diabetic with no neurological complication affecting the bladder and has not undergone instrumentation is not at greater risk of developing UTI. However, following urinary catheterisation or in the presence of an autonomic bladder the incidence of ascending infection is frequent and severe. Underlying nephrosclerosis in a diabetic kidney also increases the possibility of papillary necrosis which predisposes to infection.

Analgesic Nephropathy

This condition is associated with recurrent or asymptomatic UTI. UTI occurs in 15% to 60% of patients with analgeic nephropathy.[11] In a patient with analgesic nephropathy associated with UTI and deteriorating renal function, one has to exclude urinary tract obstruction and septicemia. The cause of urinary obstruction in a patient with analgesic nephropathy could be the result of a sloughed papilla, a calcified papilla or renal stones, transitional cell carcinoma in the renal pelvis or ureter and lastly, pyonephrosis. Analgesic nephropathy is one of the causes of sterile pyuria.

Cystitis

Acute cystitis or urethritis is common in women. An infection is termed a relapse if it occurs within 3 weeks of cessation of treatment. Reinfection accounts for about 80% of recurrent UTI. The organism is often from the perineal flora. Other foci of infection are the kidneys, prostate or the presence of any urologic abnormality. Nuns have an annual incidence of 0.4% cystitis compared to 1.6% in women aged 13 to 54 years.[12] This is because during sexual intercourse, bacteria is massaged into the urinary bladder through the anterior urethra.

E coli causes 79% of cystitis, Staph saprophyticus 11%, Klebsiella 3%, mixed organisms 3%, Proteus mirabilis 2%, enterococcus 2% and other bacteria 2%. Uropathogenetic

E coli has virulent features like increased adherence to cells, resistance to bactericidal human serum and K capsular antigen which is anti-phagocytic and causes persistent infection in a certain proportion of women with recurrent cystitis.[13]

In men, prostatic fluid itself inhibits bacterial growth and the mucus in the bladder has anti-mannose activity which discourages bacterial growth. Some females are prone to UTI because of a defect in local defence which makes them vulnerable to periurethral colonisation. This defect may be due to a lack in a particular antibody. Another reason may be the virulence of the particular strain of bacteria. Once infected, the bacteria persist.[14]

Treatment of Cystitis

The principle is to use the least toxic and least expensive antibiotic like nalidixic acid, ampicillin and nitrofurantoin. The patient should be encouraged to drink plenty of water to promote a good flow of urine to prevent urinary stasis which encourages bacterial growth. In recent years, ampicillin has been found to be less effective because of resistant strains of E coli.[13] Fifty percent of Staph saprophyticus and all Klebsiella species are now ampicillin resistant. However, augmentin which is a combination of amoxycillin and clavulinic acid is effective. The clavulinic acid destroys penicillinase produced by the bacteria and allows the amoxycillin component to act on the cell wall of the bacteria.

Nitrofurantoin is highly effective but 40% of patients experience nausea[15] Cotrimoxazole has a propensity to cause gastrointestinal upset and rash. It is also effective against Chlamydia trachomatis. The quinolones (pefloxacin, ciprofloxacin) are related to nalidixic acid and cinoxin. They are also highly effective against C trachomatis.

If a patient has symptoms of acute dysuria, suggestive of cystitis, she should be treated for UTI though the urine culture shows $<10^5$ colony counts of bacteria growth as one-third of patients with UTI has negative urine cultures.[16]

Cystitis and Urethritis

Females are 50 times more likely to have UTI than males. About 20% of females aged 24 to 60 years have at least one episode of UTI per year. After the age of 60 years the frequency is equal in both sexes.

One-third of patients with cystitis have gross haematuria. Some of these progress to upper UTI. About 40% of those with symptoms of UTI would have less than 10^5 colony counts of bacteria in the urine culture. They should still be treated as for cystitis. Fifty percent of patients with the "acute urethral syndrome" with negative cultures subsequently develop significant bacteriuria on follow-up.[16]

If urine cultures are negative for bacteria and the patient has symptoms of dysuria suggesting the urethral syndrome, one should consider C. trachomatis, N. gonorrhoea, Herpes simplex, Mycoplasma and Ureaplasma. These are organisms which cause the acute urethral syndrome. Sometimes a complaint of "dysuria" is actually due to pain caused by urine flowing over the inflamed vagina as in Candida vaginitis.

Relapsing Lower Tract Infection

In a woman with relapsing lower tract infection one should suspect an upper tract infection (pyelonephritis) and in the case of a man one should suspect prostatitis. In both sexes, a structural abnormality, stones, diverticulae should also be considered.

A patient who relapses after a week of treatment should be treated for another 2 weeks, cotrimoxazole is the best choice. If there is another relapse the patient should receive a 6-week course of treatment and an intravenous pyelogram (IVP) should be performed. Thereafter the patient should be followed up with repeat urine cultures at 2 weeks, 4 weeks, 12 weeks and 6 months to ensure eradication of the infection.

In the case of patients with chronic prostatitis they should be treated with antibiotics like cotrimoxazole, erythromycin, oleandomycin and ciprofloxacin.[17] With these antibiotics, adequate therapeutic levels can be achieved within the prostate. Treatment should be for at least 12 weeks in chronic prostatitis to ensure eradication of the infection.

Recurrent Urinary Tract Infection in the Females

Two groups of women should be considered. Those with structural or functional abnormality of the urinary tract and those with normal IVP who have lower tract infection. In some, there may be a relationship to sex or use of diaphragm but in the majority there is often no apparent cause. Infection tends to cluster in time, that is, it tends to occur more and more frequently with shorter intervals in between and then it will go off for long periods without a recurrence.

Patients should be given advice regarding sexual hygiene like voiding of the urine within 15 minutes of sexual intercourse, prolonging the period of foreplay to ensure adequate lubrication, drinking enough fluids to pass more urine to reduce urinary stasis at night and wiping from front to back to avoid introduction of perianal flora into the urethral opening.

Women with frequent lower UTI should have prophylactic antibiotics post coitally if infections are related to sex.

Nitrofurantoin one tablet post coitally is a useful prophylactic agent. Others are trimethoprim or cotrimoxazole ($\frac{1}{2}$ tablet or 240 mg) and nalidixic acid 500 mg. Women who suffer 2 or more infections a year could be taught the use of self administered single dose therapy, 4 × 480 mg of cotrimoxazole orally or 3 gm of amoxycillin or 250 mg of Ciprofloxacin orally as a single dose therapy.[18] For those who still continue to suffer recurrent UTI with prophylactic nightly antibiotics, we would prescribe suppressive therapy, either nitrofurantoin 50 mg tds, nalidixic acid 500 mg qid or cotrimoxazole 480 mg bd. This should continue for 2 years and thereafter antibiotics stopped and reinfections monitored. If reinfection occurs, it should be treated with a course of antibiotics and the suppressive regimen continued for another 2 years and then reviewed again.

Prostatitis

E coli is the commonest organism responsible for prostatitis. Others are Proteus, Klebsiella, Enterobacter, Pseudomonas and Serratia. The route of infection is

i. by ascending urethral infection
ii. reflux of infected urine into the prostatic duct and into the prostate
iii. invasion by rectal bacteria, and
iv. hematogenous route

During sexual intercourse a man can be infected by gonococcal urethritis through sexual contact with an infected female partner harbouring the gonococci in the cervix. Reflux of infected urine is another route. The presence of an indwelling catheter would enable bacteria to directly infect prostatic ducts by peri-urethral extension along the catheter. In acute prostatitis, a rectal examination will reveal a tender prostate.

Prostatic massage or instrumentation like cystoscopy should not be performed during acute prostatitis.

In a patient with prostatitis one should exclude prostatic calculi, cancer of the prostate, prostatomegaly due to benign hyperplasia and chronic prostatitis. If epididymitis is present the patient is likely to have chronic prostatitis.[17] Urethral discharge in a male could be due to urethritis, urethro-prostatitis, or prostatorrhoea (very often the result of infrequent ejaculation). Chronic bacterial prostatitis is a common cause of relapsing UTI in a male with normal IVP. If a patient has a large residual urine volume, an enlarged prostate is often the cause. In a male with positive urine cultures from mid-stream urine with no symptom of UTI, a diagnosis of prostatitis is very likely. Under these circumstances a prostatic massage should be performed. Four specimens should be obtained: void bladder urine (VBI) when urine is passed before the mid-stream urine (MSU), the mid-stream urine (VB2), expressed prostatic secretion (EPS) resulting from the massage and the fourth specimen which is the urine passed following the massage (VB3).[19,20]

Relapsing Urinary Tract Infection due to Prostatitis

Infection should be by the same pathogen with symptoms of dysuria, urgency, frequency of micturition, nocturia, suprapubic, perianal, scrotal, penile pain or hemospermia. Once treatment is stopped, symptoms recur soon after in a patient with a relapse.

Acute prostatitis should be treated for 4 to 6 weeks to prevent chronicity. Cotrimoxazole 2 tablets twice daily is a useful agent. Alternatively, one could start off with injection gentamicin plus intravenous amoxycillin for a week followed by oral cotrimoxazole once cultures confirm the sensitivity of the bacteria to the antibiotic. Other agents like erythromycin, doxycycline, cephalosporin and quinolones could be used in acute prostatitis. In acute prostatitis most antibiotics can penetrate the inflamed prostate gland because of the acute inflammation of the gland.

For chronic prostatitis treatment should be with trimethoprim, erythromycin, oleadomycin or ciprofloxacin for 12 weeks.[17] Azithromycin, the new form of Erythromycin could be used at a dose of 500 mg daily for 3 days with a break of one week. A total of 9 courses would cover 3 months. If there is no cure after 12 weeks and relapse still occurs, the infection should be treated and thereafter the patient should receive suppressive therapy with trimethoprim one tablet daily or twice daily on a long term basis for 2 years, and thereafter stopped to see if there is a relapse. If so, the patient should continue to receive therapy for another 2 years.

Non Bacterial Prostatitis

This is caused by the same organisms causing non gonococcal urethritis (NGU); apart from fungus and anaerobes. Organisms causing NGU are C. trachomatis, Ureaplasma, Mycoplasma, Trichomonads, H. simplex and Cytomegalovirus (CMV). C trachomatis causes 40% to 50% of NGU and Ureaplasma causes another 25%.[21] These organisms also cause the dysuria-pyuria syndrome where patients present with dysuria and frequency. Urine cultures should be performed to exclude gonococci and special cultures performed for C trachomatis and Ureaplasma.

Treatment for NGU consists of either erythromycin or tetracycline for 2 weeks. But in the case of non bacterial prostatitis resulting from organisms causing NGU, treatment should be for 12 weeks. Trimethoprim and ciprofloxacin could also be used. During therapy the patient should abstain from sex and alcohol. The sexual partner should also be treated. Relapse could be due to the organism becoming resistant to the antibiotic, poor patient compliance, H. simplex infection which would require therapy with iodoxyuridine or it could mean that the sexual partner has not been or has been inadequately treated.

Pregnancy

Asymptomatic bacteriuria occurs in 4% to 7% of pregnant women. About one-third of these women run the risk of developing acute pyelonephritis in the later stages of pregnancy.[22]

Screening is important as this will reduce the incidence of pyelonephritis to less than 5% in 75% of patients.[22] This will prevent the foetal morbidity due to prematurity.

In pregnancy, estrogen and progesterone induce dilatation of ureters and the renal pelvis. This will increase progressively towards term. The bladder capacity also doubles and the bladder becomes distorted due to compression by the gravid uterus.

The following antibiotics are safe in pregnancy; short acting sulphonamides, amoxycillin, nitrofurantoin and cephalosporin.[23]

Upper Urinary Tract Infection and Neurogenic Bladder

Patients with spinal cord injury require either continuous or intermittent urethral catheterisation. Renal infection is secondary to chronic upper tract infection and many patients form stones.[24]

In the past decade the use of non-sterile intermittent self catheterisation has been introduced.[25] The patients were not treated with routine prophylactic antibiotics so as to reduce incidence of emergence of resistant strains of organisms. However, others employ low dose prophylactic antibiotics with cotrimoxazole to prevent infection.[26] Continuous long term suppression with antibiotics has been used to prevent recurrent symptoms. Antibiotics used include cotrimoxazole, amoxycillin and cephalosporins.

Infection by proteus must always be suppressed as such infections predispose to stone formation which are difficult to eradicate as the bacteria lie within the stone. Some advocate treatment only for symptomatic infection. They argue against suppressive antibiotic therapy as it selects multiresistant organisms.

Catheter Associated Urinary Tract Infection

This constitutes 35% to 40% of all hospital acquired infections. It is the most common source of gram negative bacteremia. Bacteria gain entry in the following ways:

i. at time of catheterisation
ii. they enter around catheter in the urethral mucus (periurethral route)
iii. via contamination of the collecting system; bacteria ascend through the lumen of the catheter, hence the importance of using a closed drainage system

Antecedent rectal or periurethral colonisation also plays an important role as it does in female with cystitis. After a single in-out catheterisation, bacteriuria occurs in 1% of healthy persons compared to 3% to 20% among the pregnant, the elderly, debilitated and those patients with urologic abnormalities.[26]

About 50% of females and males who are catheterised for 2 weeks become bacteriuric.[26] The overall incidence increases with the duration of catheter in place and is related to the patient's condition.

Prevention of Catheter Urinary Tract Infection

The following have been advocated:

i. Closed drainage system. This prevents bacteriuria up to 10 days
ii. Twice daily application of polyantimicrobial cream to urethral meatus
iii. Systemic antibiotics in the short term not long term because this will predispose to infection with resistant strains
iv. Lubricating gels for catheter

Treatment of Catheter Urinary Tract Infection

The infected catheter should be removed, antibiotic therapy initiated and a new catheter reintroduced together with a new closed drainage system. If the patient has fever and loin pain, parenteral antibiotics should be initiated immediately and therapy continued for a week. Resistant bacteria and fungi (Candida, Torulopsis) are frequently isolated in patients on multiple courses of antibiotics. The choice of a suitable anti-fungal agent is guided by results of sensitivity tests.

Lower tract fungaria (cystitis) usually responds to amphotericin B bladder washout. First, empty the bladder of urine by means of a urinary catheter. Amphotericin B is then introduced in a dosage of 15 mg in 100 ml of distilled water through the urinary catheter. The catheter is then removed. The amphotericin will stay in the bladder and is passed out together with the urine after a few hours. Lower tract fungaria causing cystitis should respond after an amphotericin bladder wash out. After one week the urine culture should be negative for fungus. If fungus persists, it would mean that the infection is in the upper tract (pyelonephritis). If that is the case then, the patient should be treated as for an upper tract fungal infection as for systemic candidiasis (if candida is the organism grown). Intravenous amphotericin is administered following a test dose and then progressively increased until a total dosage of about 1 gm has been given, usually over a period of 6 weeks or more. Alternatively, if the organism is sensitive to 5-fluorocytosine, it could be administered intravenously for the first 2 weeks and then oral therapy given for the remaining period. This has the advantage of early discharge of the patient from hospital.

Urinary Tract Infection and the Elderly

Ageing is associated with an increased prevalence of bacteriuria. It is about 10% in males and 20% in females over the age of 65 years.[27] Young female adults have 30 times greater prevalence of bacteriuria compared to young male adults.

The following causes account for an increased prevalence of UTI in the elderly:

  i. Obstructive uropathy
 ii. Loss of bactericidal activity of prostatic secretion

iii. Poor bladder emptying due to utero-vaginal prolapse, cystocele and prostatomegaly
iv. Soiling of perineum from faeces
v. Increased bladder catheterisation

CONCLUSION

Every episode of a UTI has the potential to become a recurrent or chronic disease. Patient education is a very important aspect of the management as in many diseases which have the propensity to become chronic. Patients should be taught to anticipate subsequent episodes by teaching them to look out for early symptoms. They must understand the reasons for recurrence in order to avoid infection.

It is equally important too that the attending physician should be aware of certain aspects of the management to minimise the possibility of relapse, recurrence and chronicity. Clinical improvement does not equate bacteriologic eradication. Follow-up urine cultures are necessary to ensure cure. Depending on the circumstances of the case, whether it is a lower tract infection due to cystitis (1 week treatment), upper tract infection (2 weeks) or prostatitis (6 to 12 weeks), the physician would have to prescribe an antibiotic for varying duration. The choice of the antibiotic will depend on whether one is treating a simple recurrent cystitis in a female with normal IVP, or a patient with acute or chronic prostatitis. The choice of an antibiotic will also depend on whether it is prescribed for the current infection or for prophylactic or suppressive therapy because the emergence of multiresistant organism has to be considered. Therapy has to be accompanied by follow-up cultures and sensitivity performed at the right time and the correct periodic interval; 1 week, 2 weeks, 4 weeks, 12 weeks and 6 months to detect asymptomatic bacteriuria and at any time when the patient has a breakthrough infection.

Managed properly, the patient is likely to have a marked reduction in the incidence of relapses and recurrences, apart from the possibility of preventing a relapse or recurrence in a patient with a first or new infection. Even so, for many patients who have had a UTI, they would be prone to relapses and recurrences, often requiring long term prophylactic or suppressive antibiotics.

REFERENCES

1. White NJ, Stamm WE. eds. Cystitis and urethritis. In: Diseases of the kidney. Boston: Little Brown and Co, 1988, 1109–33.

2. Lacey RW, Lord VL, Howson GL, Luxton DEA, Trotter JC. Double blind study to compare the selection of antibiotic resistance by amoxylline or cephradine in the commensal flora. *Lancet.* 1983, **ii**:529–32.

3. Winberg J, Bollgren I, Kallenius G, Molby R, Svenson SB. Clinical pyelonephritis and focal renal scarring. *Paed Clin North Am.* 1982, **29**:801–14.

4. Woo KT. Drugs and the kidney. In: Handbook of clinical nephrology, Singapore:PG Lim Publishing 1991:182–7.

5. Sattler FR, Moyer JE, Schramm M, Lombard JS, Appelbaum PC Aztreonam compared with gentamicin for treatment of serious urinary tract infections. *Lancet.* 1984, I:1315–8.

6. Smellie JM, Ransley PG, Normand ICS, Prescod N, Edwards D. Development of new renal scars: A collaborative study. *Br Med J.* 1985, **290**:1957–60

7. Naimaldin A, Burge DM, Atwell JD. Reflux nephropathy secondary to intrauterine vesicoureteric reflux. *J Paed Surg.* 1990, **25**:287–90.

8. Bailey RR, Lynn KL, Smith AH. Long term follow-up of infants with gross vesicoureteric reflux. In: Bailey RR. ed. Second CJ Hodson Symposium on RefluxNephropathy. Christchurch, New Zealand: Typeshop, 1990:33–6.

9. Blandy JP, Singh M. The case for a more aggressive approach to staghorn calculus. *J Urol.* 1976, **115**:505–6.

10. Rous SN, Turner WR. Retrospective study of 95 patients with staghorn calculus disease. *J Urol.* 1977, **118**:902–7.

11. Murray TG, Goldberg M. Analgesic associated nephropathy in the USA: Epidemiologic, clinical and pathogenetic features. *Kidney Int.* 1978, **13**:64–71.

12. Kunin CM, McCormack RC. An epidemiological study of bacteriuria and blood pressure among nuns and working women. *N Engl J Med.* 1968, **278**:635–42.

13. Latham RH, Running K, Stamm WE. Urinary tract infections in young women caused by Staphyloccus saprophyticus. *JAMA.* 1983, **250**:3063–6.

14. Stamey TA, Fair WR, Timothy MM. Antibacterial nature of prostatic fluid. *Nature.* 1968, **218**:444–9.

15. Aronoff GR. Antimicrobial therapy for patients with renal disease. *Hosp Pract.* 1983, **18**:145–50.

16. Stamm WE, Running K, McKevitt M, Counts GW, Turk M, Holmes KK. Treatment of acute urethral syndrome. *N Engl J Med.* 1981, **304**:956–8

17. Meares EM Jr, Prostatitis: new perspectives about old woes, *J Urol.* 1980, **113**:141–7.

18. Bailey RR. Single dose therapy of urinary tract infection. In: Recent advances in Paediatrics. London: Churchill Livingstone, 1986:75–83.

19. Meares EM Jr, Stamey TA. Bacteriologic localization patterns in bacterial prostatitis and urethritis. *Invest Urol.* 1968, **5**:492–518.

20. Meares EM Jr, Barbalias GA. Prostatitis: Bacterial, nonbacterial and prostatodynia. *Semin Urol.* 1983, **1**:146–51.

21. Berger RE, Urethritis and epididymitis. *Semin Urol.* 1983, **1**:138–45.

22. Stamm WE. Prevention of urinary tract infections. *Am J Med.* 1984, **76**:148–54.

23. Zinner SH. Bacteriuria and babies revisited. *N Engl J Med.* 1979, **300**:853–5.

24. Barkin M, Dolfin D, Herschron S, Bharatwal N, Comisarow R. The urologic care of the spinal cord injury patient. *J Urol.* 1983, **129**:335–9.

25. Maynard FM, Diokno AC. Urinary infection and complications during clean intermittent catheterization following spinal cord injury. *J Urol.* 1984, **132**:943–6.

26. Krieger JN, Kaiser DL, Wenzel RP. Nosocomial urinary tract infection, secular trends, treatment and economics in a university hospital, *J Urol.* 1983, **130**:102–6.

27. Romano JM, Kaye D. Urinary tract infection in the elderly: Common yet atypical. *Geriatrics.* 1981, **36**:113–5.

CHAPTER 9

Sex and the Kidney

RELATIONSHIP BETWEEN SEXUAL INTERCOURSE AND RENAL DISEASE

The relationship between sex and the kidney has existed since the oldest profession in the world came into existence. Men who frequent brothels run the risk of infection of the urethra (urethritis) and the prostate gland (prostatitis). The infection is due to the gonococci which cause gonorrhoea. Males are infected when they have sexual intercourse with a female who harbours the infection in the cervix of her uterus without any symptoms.

One of the most feared infections is AIDS for which there is still no cure. AIDS is a disease caused by a virus called HIV, or human immuno-deficiency virus. The disease destroys part of the body's immune system, leaving victims incapable of defending themselves against infections and certain cancers. HIV is found in seminal and vaginal secretions and can be transmitted in a heterosexual or homosexual relationship.

HONEYMOON CYSTITIS

This refers to a condition in a woman who has urinary infection in the bladder following sexual intercourse. On awakening the next morning she has pain or discomfort in the bladder as well as pain each time she passes urine. There may be blood in the urine and the frequency of urination is also increased. The term "Honeymoon" refers to young brides who are at greater risk from the infection, presumably because of inexperience.

In clinical practice, however, this condition can occur in any female who has sexual intercourse. This is because in a woman the urethral opening has a very intimate relationship to the anterior wall of the vagina and both are very close to the anus. During intercourse bacteria may be introduced into the urethra thereby causing infection of the bladder. The bacteria are *Escherichia coli* which normally live in the part of the large bowel called the colon. Some are always found around the anus where they are passed out with the faeces. When the penis touches the area around the anus it picks up the bacteria which subsequently get introduced into the vagina during intercourse. When the penis contaminated with *E. coli* comes into contact with the female urethra the bacteria could then enter the urethra to cause urethritis or ascend into the bladder to cause cystitis.

What can be done for women prone to recurrent Urinary Infections?

If there is no abnormality on the IVP and if she has been engaged in sexual intercourse, then the infections are likely to be related to sexual activity.

In the case of some women, the spouse may prefer to have anal intercourse first before vaginal intercourse, thereby introducing bacteria into the urethra.

Advice on sexual hygiene is usually given to the women to prevent recurrent attacks of cystitis:

1. Empty the bladder within 15 minutes of coitus. Drink water to promote a good flow of urine to flush the organisms from the bladder.

2. Prolong the period of sexual foreplay before the actual sexual intercourse. This is especially important if either one or the other partner tends to be dry and lacking in genital lubricant. The foreplay will ensure adequate lubrication and will reduce friction and make penetration by the penis easier so that it is less likely to linger around the urethral opening to provide bacteria the opportunity of entering the urethra.

3. If adequate lubrication is not forthcoming, especially in slightly older women, then KY Jelly or other similar lubricating jelly can be applied on the genitalia. It is important not to apply too much of the jelly, otherwise the genitalia becomes too slippery and much sexual pleasure will be lost.

4. After each bowel movement wipe the anus from front to back. Similarly after passing urine wipe the area from front to back.

5. Wash with soap the area around the urethra, vagina and anus (perineum) after each bowel movement.

6. Do not use vaginal deodorants, dettol, strong soap, or antiseptic lotions for washing as they may cause irritation and inflammation of the urethra.

The doctor may prescribe an antibiotic tablet (nitrofurantoin usually) to be taken immediately after coitus. This will kill any bacteria introduced into the urethra and bladder.

In the case of a married woman who gets repeated infection many years after marriage it may be that the spouse has acquired a new preference for having anal intercourse before vaginal intercourse. The couple should be told that after anal penetration the penis should not be introduced into the vagina.

Anal Intercourse and Urinary Infection in a Male

A male who practises anal intercourse with a woman may himself sometimes get urinary tract infection because bacteria from her anus could find their way into his urethra and from there into the bladder. Usually, however, this is uncommon as bacteria in the male urethra is also flushed out with the emission of semen. Moreover the long male urethra also makes ascending infection less likely.

Oral Intercourse and Urinary Infection

Usually this is uncommon as saliva from the woman's mouth itself inhibits bacterial activity. However vigorous oral activity by the female may cause a soreness at the urethral opening. Occasionally, there may be minor trauma at the urethral opening which could be infected giving rise to pain on passing urine.

Urinary Tract Infection in Sexy Young Males

Until recently, UTI in young men was believed to be confined to those with an underlying abnormality of the urinary tract. It is now recognised that uncomplicated cystitis can occur in young men and "can even mimic urethritis". Risk factors include anal intercourse, HIV infection, lack of circumcision, having a sexual partner with colonization of the vagina with uropathogens. Seven day treatment regimen are usually adequate and imaging is only necessary in those who fail to respond to therapy. Prostatitis have to be considered in those who fail to respond to therapy or have recurrent infection.

Reference:
E.G Smyth and N O'Connell. Complicated urinary tract infection. Current Opinion in Infections Diseases, 1998, 11 (1) : 63–66.

In a woman who has repeated bruising to the urethral opening following Sexual Intercourse what could be done?

Varying the position of sexual intercourse may avoid bruising. One way is to have intercourse with the male penetrating the female from a posterior position. This way, the urethral opening is spared from friction but the female may suffer discomfort from pressure on the bladder. Emptying the bladder before coitus will help.

Significance of Blood Stained Semen

When a male ejaculates, sometimes the seminal fluid may be blood stained. The commonest cause is an infection of the urinary bladder (cystitis or prostatitis). He should seek medical treatment as he may require investigation if he does not respond to a course of antibiotics.

Impotency

Impotency is the term used when a male is incapable of performing the sexual act. Impotency occurs with increasing frequency over the age of 40, affecting 50% of males in their late sixties. In most cases no organic explanation can be found. The younger man may require psychiatric evaluation. Systemic disease like diabetes, causing diabetic autonomic neuropathy and drugs given for hypertension and specific neurological problems should be excluded. Measurement of hormone levels and hormonal treatment are usually not very useful.

Causes of Impotency

There are many causes of impotency:

- Psychological.
- Injury or tumours in the brain (especially temporal lobe).
- Spinal cord injury or tumours.
- Drugs which depress the brain (barbiturates, alcohol).
- Drugs which block the action of nerves, especially drugs used in the treatment of hypertension (guanethidine, bethanidine, methyldopa, clonidine and some beta adrenergic blocking drugs).
- Interference with blood supply to lower part of body: disease and narrowing of blood vessels due to arteriosclerosis (aorto-iliac arteriosclerosis, bilateral lumbar sympathectomy).
- Inappropriate hormones: lack of male hormones (androgen) or excessive female hormones (oestrogen).

CHAPTER 10

Hypertension and the Kidney

CAUSES OF HYPERTENSION

1. Essential hypertension.
2. Renal parenchymal causes are acute and chronic glomerulonephritis (GN), chronic pyelonephritis, diabetic nephropathy, lupus nephritis, obstructive uropathy and polycystic kidneys. Other causes are systemic sclerosis, haemolytic uraemic syndrome and haemangiopericytoma.
3. Renovascular causes are renal artery stenosis due to atheromatous changes, fibromuscular dysplasia, Takayasu's disease or hypoplastic kidneys.
4. Endocrine causes are Cushing's syndrome, Conn's syndrome, phaeochromocytoma, carcinoid syndrome, hyperparathyroidism.
5. Drug induced causes: Eg. oral contraceptives, liquorice, corticosteroids, prostaglandin synthetase inhibitors, monoamine oxidase inhibitors.
6. Others: coarctation of the aorta, toxaemia of pregnancy.

RENAL EFFECTS OF HYPERTENSION

1. Hypertension decreases renal plasma flow.
2. When hypertension is uncontrolled, glomerular filtration is impaired. This will cause glomerulosclerosis. With time renal impairment occurs.

3. Deterioration of renal function is especially rapid in patients with malignant hypertension or accelerated hypertension.

4. Malignant hypertension (diastolic BP > 120 mm Hg with presence of papilloedema) can complicate hypertension due to whatever cause. This includes patients with benign essential hypertension. Hence it is very important to ensure that hypertension is well controlled at all times. This is especially so among patients with glomerular disease as uncontrolled hypertension accelerates the progression of glomerular lesions causing diffuse sclerosing glomerulonephritis.

INVESTIGATION OF THE PATIENT WITH HYPERTENSION

History

Take a thorough history of the disease, its onset, how well the control has been and whether the patient was compliant with his medication. Very often there is no preceding history which could provide a clue to the cause of hypertension. A history of urinary abnormalities some years ago may point to glomerulonephritis as the cause. Paroxysms or symptoms related to sympathetic overactivity may alert one to the possibility of phaeochromocytoma. Flushing of the face with diarrhoea may be a clue to carcinoid syndrome.

Enquire about a family history of hypertension, diabetes mellitus or kidney disease (polycystic kidneys, hereditary nephritis). A strong family history of hypertension makes the diagnosis of essential hypertension more likely. Ask about drug history. In women, a history of oral contraceptive usage is important. Was there a history of toxaemia of pregnancy?

Physical Examination

1. In addition to routine examination, look for evidence of end organ damage due to hypertension — left ventricle hypertrophy, heart failure, changes of hypertensive retinopathy on fundoscopy (Keith and Wagner's grading I to IV; look for macular star as it is associated with renal insufficiency), cerebral vascular insufficiency and atherosclerosis of peripheral blood vessels.
2. Check for delayed femoral pulses and prominent collateral circulation as it points to coarctation of the aorta. Absent radial pulse and vascular bruits in the neck may be clues for a diagnosis of Takayasu's disease.
3. Listen for an abdominal bruit which would indicate renal artery stenosis.
4. Certain conditions like Cushing's syndrome or carcinoid syndrome will be diagnosed more easily when the physical signs are obvious. Enquire about steroid therapy in a patient with features of Cushing's.
5. Patients who have stigmata of systemic lupus erythematosus often have characteristic facies due to steroid therapy or because of the erythematosus rash on the face, or evidence of vasculitis and Raynaud's phenomenon.
6. Stigmata of chronic renal failure will not be missed if one remembers renal failure as a cause of hypertension.

Investigation

1. Urine microscopy and cultures.
2. Full blood count.
3. Blood urea and serum creatinine.
4. Serum electrolytes. Hypokalaemic alkalosis in a hypertensive, not treated with diuretics, should alert one to the possibility of Conn's syndrome.

5. Fasting blood glucose to exclude diabetes mellitus because diabetics have a higher incidence of hypertension and diabetic nephropathy has to be excluded.
6. Serum calcium. Hypercalcaemia is a cause of hypertension and a cause of acute hypercalcaemia should be looked for.
7. Creatinine clearance to assess renal function and total urinary proteinuria to exclude renal disease.
8. Urinary VMA (vanillyl-mandelic acid) and catecholamines should be measured in a young hypertensive to exclude phaeochromocytoma.
9. Five HIAA (hydroxy indole acetic acid) to exclude carcinoid syndrome.
10. ECG, Chest X-ray are necessary to assess cardiac status.
11. Intravenous pyelogram may be necessary if renal disease is suspected.

Special Investigations

1. Plasma renin assay is essential in the investigation of a patient with hypokalaemic alkalosis associated with hypertension. A low plasma renin activity (PRA) may indicate Conn's syndrome. A high PRA may indicate ischaemic renal lesions. Computerised axial tomography is valuable in the assessment of a patient suspected to have adrenal masses.
2. If renal artery stenosis is suspected as a cause of hypertension, a rapid sequence IVP or a DTPA radio-isotope scan can be performed to demonstrate the decreased perfusion on the side with the stenotic artery. The kidney with the stenotic artery is smaller then the normal side by at least 1.5 cm. The nephrogram is faint, the pyelographic phase is delayed, but there is increased concentration of the contrast on the delayed film. However, both techniques fail to detect 20% to 30% of proven cases of renal artery

stenosis. A renal arteriogram is the most diagnostic procedure for renal artery stenosis.

3. The plasma renin activity can be used to predict blood pressure response to surgery. PRA from the renal veins and the peripheral veins have to be sampled. A clear gradient of PRA between the renal vein and the peripheral vein as well as suppression of renin activity from the uninvolved kidney indicates that the stenotic side is the cause of the hypertension and response to surgery is good.

4. Saralasin (a competitive antagonist of angiotensin II) infusion test is another useful way of establishing that the blood pressure is angiotensin dependent. A fall of diastolic blood pressure of 10 mm Hg in response to saralasin predicts good response to surgery.

5. Captopril Test: an ACE inhibitor eliminates Angiotensin II induced glomerular arteriolar vasoconstriction. In the kidney with renal artery stenosis, a decrease in renal function (GFR) is seen after captopril administration. Captopril is given in an oral dose of 50 mg and the radiopharmaceutical used in the renogram is Technetium (Tc)-99m DTPA or Tc-99m MAG3. A routine (pre-captopril) renal scan is performed. This is followed 4 to 48 hours later with a second scan performed after administration of captopril (post-captropril scan). Some institutions perform post captopril scan first. If it is normal, the study is stopped.

TREATMENT OF RENAL ARTERY STENOSIS

1. Anti-hypertensive drugs are the first line of management.
2. If hypertension proves difficult to control, percutaneous transluminal angioplasty (PTCA) with a balloon catheter should be performed.
3. Surgery is resorted to if PTCA fails. Bypass procedures can be performed, especially in bilateral renal artery stenosis.

Autotransplantation of the affected kidney has also been successful in selected cases.

4. If there is hardly any function left in the stenosed kidney, as in the case of segmental hypoplasia, nephrectomy can be performed.

Medical Management of Hypertension

There is a need to monitor the serum cholesterol, control obesity, reduce salt intake and stop smoking.

1. Endocrine causes of hypertension are identified and treated.
2. There are at least 7 main groups of hypotensive agents which can be employed in the treatment of hypertension, viz:

i)   Diuretics (see chapter on Diuretics)
     A diuretic can be used for mild hypertension.
ii) Beta Blockers
     Beta Blockers can be classified as follows:

• Non-specific	— propranolol
• Cardioselective	
— produce less bronchoconstriction	— metoprolol, atenolol
• Alpha Beta Blocker	
— postural hypotension is more common because of alpha blockade	— labetalol
• Intrinsic sympathomometic	
— useful for those with compromised cardiac function	— pindolol, oxyprenolol
• Renal vasodilating	
— increases renal blood flow	— nadolol tertatolol

iii)   Alpha Blocker (prazosin, phentolamine, labetalol)
iv)   Smooth muscle relaxants (hydrallazine, minoxidil, nitroprusside, diazoxide, indapamide)
Vasodilators tend to cause fluid retention and is usually combined with a diuretic.
Minoxidil causes hirsutism and is best avoided in females.
v)   Calcium Antagonists (nifedipine, amlodipine)
Only long acting Nifedipine should be used as the short acting preparation has been reported to cause episodic rises in BP associated with significant morbidity.
However, given sublingually, short acting Nifedipine is useful for quick and effective control of severe hypertension. Some patients however cannot tolerate nifedipine because of severe giddiness and flushing with headaches.
Longer acting ones like Adalat LA is preferred. Another useful long acting calcium channel blocker or calcium ion antagonist is Amlodipine (Norvasc) which has minimal side effects like headaches and palpitations.
vi)   Angiotensin Converting Enzyme (ACE) Inhibitor (captopril, enalapril)
This is a class of anti-hypertensives which inhibits conversion of angiotensin I to angiotensin II. Its side effects consist of taste disturbances, cough, skin rash and when high doses are combined with immuno-suppressive agents, as in patients with lupus nephritis, leucopenia and agranulocytosis may occur. When using captopril, one should start with a small test dose (6.25 mg) at night to assess the initial response to the drug as there may be severe postural hypotension. This is more likely to happen in those patients who are volume depleted. Enalapril which is a long acting ACE inhibitor is an easier drug to use.
ACE inhibitors may cause acute renal failure. This is due to relief of angiotensin II dependent vasoconstriction of the glomeruli's efferent arterioles, resulting in decrease

in intraglomerular BP and therefore decreased GFR, hence the renal failure. The renal failure is reversible with cessation of ACE Inhibitor therapy. Caution should therefore be exercised in patients with renal impairment as the renal function may worsen further. Reversible renal failure also occurs when ACE inhibitor is used to treat patients with hypertension with a single kidney. In fact, this principle is used as a test for the presence of renal artery stenosis in a transplant patient with hypertension as such a patient will have renal impairment on being treated with ACE inhibitor. Monitor the serum creatinine and serum K^+ of patients with renal impairment who are on ACE Inhibitors. Hyperkalaemia is due to the anti-Aldosterone effect of ACE inhibitor.

vii) Angiotensin II receptor antagonist (Losartan, valsartan, candesartan). This is a new class of anti-hypertensives which binds selectively to the Angiotensin receptor, thus preventing the binding of angiotensin II at the receptor site. It blocks all physiologically relevant actions of Angiotensin II. Its renoprotective effects in conditions associated with glomerular hyperfiltration is similar to ACE inhibitors. Like ACE inhibitors its side effects include acute renal failure and hyperkalaemia. It is useful in patients who cannot agree with ACE inhibitors due to the side effect of cough.

It is important to remember that in long standing hypertension, autoregulation of blood flow to major organs is impaired. If blood pressure in these patients is brought down too rapidly, the perfusion to a vital organ may drop so drastically as to result in impaired function. This will explain renal deterioration in some patients who have their hypertension suddenly too well controlled.

In certain situations it is absolutely important to control hypertension rapidly. These are:

1. Dissecting aneurysm
2. Hypertensive encephalopathy
3. Eclampsia of pregnancy
4. Subarachnoid haemorrhage associated with hypertension
5. Malignant hypertension with rapidly deteriorating renal function

Drugs Used in Emergency Treatment of Hypertension

1. Sublingual short acting nifedipine (10 mg, repeated 4 hourly)
2. Injection Hydrallazine (I.V. or I.M. 50 mg)
3. Nitroprusside (continuous infusion)

ROLE OF SODIUM AND POTASSIUM IN HYPERTENSION

Story of Evolution

Man over the last million years consumed only 5% of the sodium we now eat. He was a forager and ate mainly vegetable which contained large amounts of potassium. Three hundred to four hundred years ago, salt became readily available from the sea and salt mines. Salt was found to have the magical property of preserving food. Today, because of instinctive appetite and the easy availability of processed food, we are used to eating large amounts of salt in our diet.

Sodium and Blood Pressure

Communities with a high salt intake have an increased risk of developing hypertension. Primitive communities which eat less salt and have a higher potassium intake have a lower risk of developing hypertension. The sodium/potassium ratio in the diet is a better determinant of blood pressure than either sodium or potassium alone.

How does Salt Raise Blood Pressure?

The abnormality causing hypertension is believed to reside in the kidney and patients with essential hypertension have difficulty in excreting sodium. Professor HE de Wardener and GA MacGregor think they have an inherited defect to get rid of sodium *(Kidney International* 1980, 18:1–9).

A high sodium intake increases the secretion of natriuretic hormone. This hormone causes the kidney to excrete sodium. But at the same time natriuretic hormone also inhibits the sodium pumps (sodiumpotassium ATPase) in the smooth muscle cells of the arterioles. This in turn leads to an increase in intracellular calcium which causes increased contractility of the arteriole smooth muscle, giving rise to increased peripheral resistance and hence hypertension.

Does Salt Restriction Lower Blood Pressure?

There is considerable evidence that severe reduction of sodium intake lowers raised blood pressure. The Kempner rice and fruit diet which has low sodium and protein and high potassium has also been shown to lower blood pressure in hypertensive individuals. MacGregor conducted a study on 19 patients *(Lancet* 1982, 1:351–354) in a double blind trial where sodium intake was reduced by half (160 mmol/day to 80 mmol/day) for 2 weeks, and documented a fall in blood pressure of the patients with reduced sodium intake.

Role of Potassium

Potassium is also important in blood pressure regulation. In the 1930s it was used as a diuretic. Even then there was already a suggestion that increasing potassium intake might lower blood pressure. In rats, increasing the intake of potassium blunts the effects of sodium on blood pressure and this can prevent a rise of blood pressure due to high sodium intake.

MacGregor in a study of 23 patients *(Lancet* 1986, II:567–570) in a double blind crossover trial of slow K versus placebo, where patients were given 8 slow K tablets per day (64 mmols of K^+) reported that patients given slow K had a small but significant fall in blood pressure.

Presently patients with hypertension (and normal renal function) are urged to increase potassium intake by taking more fruits and vegetables. Oranges, banana and skim milk are useful sources of potassium. Experimentally, rats given a high potassium diet were protected from blood vessel lesions of hypertension in the brain, heart and kidney in spite of raised blood pressure whereas control rats not on a high potassium diet had the vascular lesions of hypertension.

Essential Hypertension: A Renal Perspective

There is now evidence that essential hypertension results from an inherited renal tendency towards excessive vasoconstriction or an inability to appropriately increase renal blood flow. Studies of African-Americans show that their hypertension is seen at an earlier age, increases more quickly with time, has a higher prevalence, is more severe and is associated with more adverse cardiovascular and renal effects; excluding primary atherosclerotic disease (Hypertension 1993; 21: 380–90).

Recently Johnson and Schreiner (Kidney International, 1997, 52: 1169–79) — hypothesized that Essential Hypertension is a form of Acquired Tubulointerstitial Disease. The Hypothesis is that HPT is a 2 phase disease. The first phase is episodic HPT which is due to a Hyperactive Renin Angiotensin and Sympathetic Nervous System. Later on, a second phase sets in whereby there is persistent hypertension due to an inability to excrete salt. What causes people with 1st Phase Hypertension to develop 2nd Phase Hypertension or established Essential Hypertension, that is, the transition from the 1st to the 2nd Phase is the result of catecholamine induced interstitial disease. Excess catecholamine due to over- stimulation of the Sympathetic Nervous System causes increased peritubular capillary pressure and a reduction of peritubular capillary blood flow causing preferential ischaemia in the juxta-medullary region since it does not antoregulate well to changes in renal perfusion pressure. This causes local injury to the tubulo-interstitium and peritubular capillary which triggers the release of vasoconstrictors (angiotensin II, adenosine) and inhibition of vasodilators (nitric oxide, prostaglandins, dopamine) that further augment ischemia. The end result of this injury is that there is an increase in Tubulo-Glomerular (TG) Feedback with enhanced NaCl resorption and blunting of Pressure Natriuresis (PN) with decreased NaCl excretion. The combined effect of increased TG feedback and decreased of PN leads to defective NaCl excretion with persistent Hypertension. What happens is that ischemia of the tubulo-interstitium with time leads to Glomerular Hyperfiltration and proteinuria and finally chronic renal failure. The proteinuria in patients with Essential Hypertension is a sign of Acquired Tubulo-Interstitial

Disease. It also explains why patients with Essential Hypertension develop renal failure. Hence Essential Hypertension is no longer held to be a benign disease. In the past it was thought that, as long as BP was well controlled a patient with Essential Hypertension will not develop kidney failure. But this is no longer so. There are studies in patients with Hypertension which show that a significant number of patients do develop chronic renal failure. The classical example is in the African-American in the USA where there is a high incidence of ESRF due to Hypertensive Nephosclerosis. In a study in UK (QJM, 1993; 86: 271–275) by Innes et al, among 185 renal biopsies (2.5% of 7339 biopsies) with Benign Nephrosclerosis due to Essential Hypertension, more than 1.5 gm of proteinuria occurred in 40% of patients. Seven had Nephrotic Range Proteinuria, 25% had microscopic hamaturia, 51% had renal impairment. All these 185 patients had long standing Essential Hypertension, none with co-existing renal disease.

In Singapore we estimate the incidence of Hypertensive Nephrosclerosis is at least 9%. The incidence of new ESRF patients in Singapore is about 550 a year, 9% would mean about 50 patients a year.

CHAPTER 11

Diuretics

Diuretics are useful agents and are indicated for patients with oedema due to salt and water retention from various causes. They are also popular as therapy for patients with mild hypertension or as an adjunct to other hypotensive agents. This chapter discusses the action and side effects of diuretics and their role in the treatment of hypertension.

Diuretics can cause disorder in acid-base balance as well as disturbances in fluid and electrolyte balance. Before prescribing diuretics to a patient one must always enquire about a history of diabetes mellitus or gout as diuretics can worsen these conditions. Potassium losing diuretics can also cause hypokalaemia in patients on digoxin which may precipitate arrhythmias.

A patient on diuretics should be assessed regularly with regards to his volume status and sodium stores to make sure he is not dehydrated or salt depleted. Baseline data like blood urea, electrolytes, uric acid and calcium should be obtained before commencing treatment. Similarly the lipid profile of the patient should also be ascertained. This is because diuretics can cause derangement in these parameters.

Thiazides

1. Thiazides inhibit sodium chloride (NaCl) reabsorption in the distal convoluted tubule of the kidneys. It has a second

site of action in the proximal tubule when combined with a loop diuretic (see Fig. 11.1).

2. There is an active reabsorptive process for calcium in the distal convoluted tubule. Thiazides augment this action and cause hyper-calcaemia. This is the result of a sodium/calcium exchange system plus an ATP-dependent calcium pump.

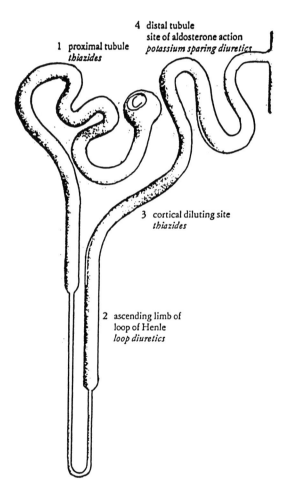

Fig. 11.1   Sites of action of diuretics

3. Thiazides also have an extra-renal action causing vasodilatation of blood vessels and thereby achieving a mild blood pressure lowering effect.

Side Effects of Thiazide Diuretic

1. It causes weakness, fatigue, impotency and paresthesia.
2. Potassium depletion; metabolic alkalosis due to volume contraction and secondary aldosteronism.
3. Hypokalaemia causes ventricular ectopics.
4. Leads to decreased insulin secretion and impaired glucose tolerance test.
5. Causes elevation of total cholesterol, low density lipoprotein (LDL) cholesterol and triglycerides and predisposes the patient to atheroma formation.
6. Elevation of uric acid.
7. Causes hyponatraemia and dehydration if given in excess.
8. Causes hypomagnesaemia which can induce arrhythmia.
9. Causes hypercalcaemia.
10. Occasionally, patients may be allergic to thiazides, developing skin rash, haemolytic anaemia, thrombocytopenia, acute pancreatitis, jaundice and interstitial nephritis.

Loop Diuretic (Frusemide, Ethacrynic Acid, Bumetamide)

1. Inhibits NaCl reabsorption in thick ascending limb at the loop of Henle.
2. Side effects are hypokalaemic metabolic alkalosis, magnesium wasting, hypercalcaemia and ototoxicity.
3. Other side effects include hypersensitivity, myelo-suppression, skin rash, liver dysfunction, paresthesia and interstitial nephritis.

4. Combined with thiazide, both agents increase NaCl delivery out of the proximal tubule.
5. Bumetamide is more potent on a weight to weight basis. 1 mg of bumetamide = 40 mg of frusemide. It has an additional site of action at the proximal tubule. All loop diuretics produce diuresis even in severe renal failure, but high doses have to be used.

Spironolactone (Aldactone)

1. It antagonises the action of aldosterone at the distal tubule thereby preventing the reabsorption of sodium.
2. Its main side effect is hyperkalaemia as it is a potassium sparing diuretic.
3. Should be used with caution in patients with renal impairment. These patients tend to have hyperkalaemia since potassium is retained in renal failure. Caution is needed in prescribing spironolactone to patients on potassium supplements as there is a risk of hyperkalaemia.
4. Monitor electrolytes for hyperkalaemia.

Indapamide (Natrilix)

1. This is an indoline derivative of chlorosulphonamide with both diuretic and anti-hypertensive activity.
2. It has a mild diuretic action at the distal tubule, and a vasodilator action due to a direct inhibitory action on smooth muscle stimulated by noradrenaline and angiotensin II by reducing transmembrane calcium current.
3. It is more active than spironolactone and frusemide in inhibiting thromboxane A2 and stimulates prostacycline to a greater extent than frusemide.
4. Its extra-renal anti-hypertensive effect is useful in patients with renal failure and it does not have the dose-related side effects of thiazide in the treatment of hypertension.

5. Given in a small dose of 2.5 *mg* a day, it has only mild diuretic but significant vasodilator hypotensive effect. If the dose is doubled or if given twice a day the diuretic effect becomes more manifest. Long acting Indapamide is also available.

Diuretic Therapy and Vascular Disease

1. What is the net effect of diuretic therapy on risk factors for vascular disease?
2. Ames (1983) and the Framingham data *(Annals New York Academy of Science* 1963, 107:539–556) showed that though diuretics lower BP, they also increase serum cholesterol and impair glucose tolerance test. The probability of developing vascular disease increased from 7.8% to 8.6%. Morgan (1980) showed that patients with mild hypertension on diuretics had a mortality double that predicted and the incidence of myocardial infarction increased 3 fold.

Beta Blockers and Cardiac Protection

1. Beta blockers are associated with raised total and LDL cholesterol, triglycerides and decreased HDL cholesterol — factors promoting atheroma.
2. However, this is counterbalanced by cardio-protective effect of beta blockers.
3. Beta blockers reduce cardiovascular morbidity and mortality following myocardial infarction.

Comparison of Beta Blocker and Diuretic

1. There is no difference in the degree of control of BP.

2. In the control of mild hypertension, diuretic causes impotency, gout and glucose intolerance, whereas beta blockers cause cold extremities, breathlessness and lethargy.

3. One may therefore decide to choose the drug on the basis of side effects. It is probably safe to use diuretics for mild hypertension provided the patient has normal lipid profiles. These profiles will have to be monitored periodically while the patient is on treatment with diuretics.

Current Role of Diuretics in Hypertension

1. There is general agreement that diuretics are of value in the treatment of hypertension in spite of the potential side effects. They should probably be used as first line therapy in the elderly.

2. Low dose diuretic has less side effect, eg. 12.5 mg hydrochlorthiazide. If this proves effective it may regain its role as the drug of choice.

3. For a young patient, some may consider a beta blocker as a first line treatment, a vasodilator as second line and low dose diuretic as a third line, especially since vasodilators also cause fluid retention.

4. Angiotensin Converting Enzyme (ACE) inhibitors are also particularly effective with diuretics.

5. Angiotensin Receptor Antagonist (ATRA) are also more effective with diuretics.

6. Though diuretics may have lost the number one place to vasodilators as the choice therapy for hypertension, they still play, an important role in the treatment of the disease, especially when combined with a hypotensive drug.

7. There is a place for low dose diuretics which do not cause biochemical cardiovascular risk or impotence.

Treatment of Renal Hypertension

1. Treatment of hypertension in patients with renal insufficiency reduces morbidity and mortality and helps to arrest the progression of renal damage.
2. Use beta blockers, calcium channel blockers, ACE inhibitors, or ATRA.
3. When GFR < 25 ml/min, thiazides are usually ineffective.
4. Potassium sparing diuretics are dangerous and loop diuretics are preferred.
5. An alternative is indapamide.

Treatment of Essential Hypertension

1. For mild essential hypertension, thiazide is used provided patient has normal lipid profile. Adequate control is obtained in two-thirds of patients.

2. If there is no response, use a beta blocker, calcium channel blocker, ACE inhibitor or ATRA. Salt and water retention may be a consequence of a calcium channel blocker or vasodilator.

3. Thiazide also has a direct effect on vascular smooth muscle causing vasodilatation.

4. Borderline hypertensives respond to salt load with rise in BP. A diuretic may be useful. Thiazide may be preferred as it has a 12 to 18 hours' duration of action.

5. There is however, the problem of renal potassium wasting due to diuretic induced potassium depletion which may give rise to ventricular ectopy. Dietary potassium supplement or oral potassium chloride is necessary. Check renal function to exclude renal impairment before prescribing potassium chloride supplements.

6. Alternatively, one could use potassium sparing diuretics like triamterene or diazide (a combination of triamterene plus thiazide). Triamterene and amiloride (also a potassium sparing diuretic) inhibit entry of sodium into the distal tubule and collecting duct by acting directly at the mucosal surface. However, triamterene has its side effects. It is associated with renal calculi (Ettinger, 1980). Among 181 renal calculi (0.4% or 56 000 calculi), 1/3 contained mainly triamterene. It also causes birefringent crystals and brownish casts which resemble granular casts in urine (Fairley 1983, Fairley and Woo, *Clinical Nephrology* 1986, 26:169–173). The casts can be differentiated from true granular casts as they show birefringence when examined under the microscope using polarised light. Presumably, the formation of triamterene casts is a predisposing factor to calculi formation. In addition, Triamterene may be associated with anuric renal failure as experimentally, the site of formation of triamterene casts in the rat was mainly in the medullary and papillary collecting ducts. Its other side effects are interstitial nephritis and nephrotoxicity especially with NSAID.

7. Beta blockers are often the first step in the treatment of essential hypertension in the United Kingdom, Scandinavia and the United States. However, others may prefer to start treatment with calcium channel blocker to avoid the side effects of beta blockers altogether. Alternatively, some may choose an ACE inhibitor like enalapril, or an Angiotensin Receptor Antagonist.

Tailor Treatment to Patient

1. Whatever the mode of therapy, one should always tailor the treatment to the patient. For young patients with high sympathetic activity and high plasma renin activity (PRA), they may respond better to a beta blocker.

2. For the old patients with low PRA, a diuretic may be preferable as they are more prone to the side effects of beta blockers like congestive heart failure and peripheral ischaemia.

3. Old patients with low PRA may respond well to calcium antagonists.

4. Small doses of ACE inhibitors or ATRA are also useful in the elderly. Check renal function and serum potassium.

CHAPTER 12

Kidney Stones

THE INCIDENCE OF STONE DISEASE

In Britain and Scandinavia, the incidence of stone disease is 0.2 to 0.5 per 1000 in the population. In Thailand it is 8 per 1000. The Central and South American Indians, Bantus and Black races in the United States are somehow protected from stone disease. Stone disease is commoner in dry climates and where people sweat a lot, especially among individuals who allow themselves to get dehydrated and not drink enough water to replace the fluid loss.

In Singapore, stones are twice as common in males than in females. It seems to be commoner among doctors. Location wise, 42% of stones are found in the kidney, 49% in the ureters, 7% in the bladder and 2% in the urethra. The peak incidence is from 20 to 40 years. 12.5% of patients experience recurrences and about one-third lose a kidney. (Data by courtesy of K.T. Foo)

FACTORS WHICH PREDISPOSE TO STONE FORMATION

1. The pH of urine affects stone formation. Eg. uric acid stones form in acidic urine.
2. Stones form when there is a high concentration of certain stone forming substances in the urine. If the concentration of these substances rises to a certain level stones are

formed. If there is a lot of water in the urine to dilute these substances there is a lesser chance of stones forming. This explains why people who sweat a lot and do not drink enough water have a tendency to form stones.

3. We have certain naturally occurring inhibitors in the urine which prevent stones from forming. Some people have less of these substances and are therefore more prone to stones.

4. Other factors such as obstruction to the free flow of urine causing stasis predisposes a person to stone formation. Infection by certain urea splitting bacteria can also cause stone formation.

THE DIFFERENT TYPES OF STONES

90% of renal stones are principally of calcium salts (calcium oxalate, calcium phosphate). A small proportion of these are composed of calcium, magnesium ammonium phosphate or triple phosphates which have a tendency to form 'Staghom' stones. The Staghorn calculi predisposes to infection and obstruction.

The remaining 10% of renal stones are uric stones. People living in hot climate who sweat a lot and drink little water tend to form uric acid stones.

35% of all stones among Singaporeans contain uric acid; 10% as urates alone and 25% in association with triple phosphates.

SYMPTOMS OF STONES IN THE URINARY TRACT

Many people have kidney stones but are often not aware of it until they develop symptoms. 75% of patients may complain of pain or backache, others may pass blood in the urine (31%) or have urinary tract infections (14%) and yet others may have the stones diagnosed on X-ray for some unrelated complaint (5%).

Pain due to kidney stone is called "renal colic". Actually this pain is felt only when the stone is moving down the ureter. The colic or pain results from contraction of the muscles in the ureter as it tries to force the stone lower down the ureter in an attempt to expel it. The pain usually starts in the left or right side of the abdomen and travels towards the groin and may radiate to the testicle in the case of males. It can be a very severe pain causing the patient to double up in bed or toss about in agony.

Large stones that are too big to be passed down the ureter can cause obstruction (7%) giving rise to a dull ache in the back. Bladder stones can sometimes cause a dragging sensation. When passing urine the stone may act like a ball valve causing urine to start, stop and start again. In addition there may be pain in the penis, bloody urine or bladder infection causing the patient frequent pain on passing urine.

INVESTIGATION OF PATIENTS WITH STONES

1. Urine is examined for presence of blood or infection caused by stones.
2. Blood tests are performed to check kidney function (blood urea and creatinine). Blood calcium and uric acid levels are also checked as high blood calcium or blood uric acid forms stones.
3. X-rays of the abdomen or intravenous pyelogram (IVP) are done to determine the site and number of stones. An ultrasound investigation is also useful to identify the site of the stone and exclude obstruction.

4. If it is suspected that the stone has caused obstruction to the flow of urine, a tube is passed into the bladder (cystoscopy) and through it fine catheters are passed up to the ureters. Contrast dye is injected and X-ray pictures are taken to demonstrate the site of obstruction.
5. 24 hours' urine is collected to measure calcium and uric acid in the urine. Excessive amounts of calcium and uric acid in the urine can cause kidney stones.
6. Stones passed out should be sent for stone analysis to determine the type of stone.

TREATMENT OF PATIENT WITH RENAL STONES

1. There are certain medical conditions which cause stones to form in the kidney. If these conditions are treated or removed then further stones will not form.
2. It is important that patients who have stones in the kidney should drink plenty of water to maintain a high urine volume as this will lower the concentration of substances which cause stones to form or even dissolve existing stones. Patients should drink enough water to pass at least 3 litres of urine a day. The patient should drink water before going to bed so that he would get up in the night to pass urine. After passing, he should drink (from the tumbler of water by the bedlocker) before lying in bed so that he would wake again to pass urine. Initially he may be apprehensive of broken or lost sleep but after a while he will get used to the waking process and having no difficulty in automatically falling asleep again. He will not therefore suffer from insomnia.
3. Stones that are less than 0.5 cm in diameter can be passed out but those more than 0.5 cm will require surgical intervention.
4. If the patient has severe pain he can be given an injection to relieve the pain.

5. Urinary infection can be treated with antibiotics.
6. Recurrent stones due to excessive amounts of calcium in the urine can be treated with chlorothiazide (a diuretic). This will decrease the incidence of recurrence. In addition the patient should avoid high calcium food like dairy products (milk and cheese). Those who have stones due to too much uric acid in the urine can be treated with allopurinol which is also used for the treatment of gout. In addition, these patients also require alkalinisation of their urine by taking sodium bicarbonate solution and avoidance of food containing high urate content (liver, kidney and other organ meat).
7. Stones that cannot be passed out and give rise to severe pain, urine infection or bleeding into the urine will require surgery.

Newer Techniques of Stone Removal

1. Percutaneous Nephrolithotomy (PCN)

This involves making a tract (tunnel) from the skin to the kidney. An instrument called a nephroscope is introduced to view the stone in the kidney. A small stone is removed by means of a pair of forceps passed through the nephroscope. A large stone is broken up by means of ultrasound and then removed with forceps or sucked out.

2. Extracorporeal Shock Wave Lithotripsy (ESWL)

The patient is immersed in a water bath and an external source of shock waves, generated by means of an electrode and a generator, is focussed on the stone in the kidney to cause it to break up. The fragments of stone are then passed out in the urine.

3. *Transurethral Urethroscopy*

Preliminary dilatation of the vesico-ureteric junction with ureteric bougies or balloon catheter is made. A ureteroscope is then introduced to view the stone which is then removed. Larger stones are disintegrated by ultrasound before removal.

GOUT

Gout is a condition due to excess uric acid in the blood which occasionally crystallises out into the joints giving rise to very severe pain, usually in the big toe. The toe becomes red, swollen and acutely tender. Attacks of gout often come on at night or in the early hours of the morning.

What Triggers Off an Attack of Gout?

A heavy meal containing too much offal (liver, kidneys, fish roe), heavy wine, undue exertion, an operation or severe illness; anything which suddenly changes the patient's lifestyle can precipitate an attack of gout. Such attacks may therefore occur more commonly on holidays or during travel overseas.

Treatment of Gout

The acute attack can be treated with either colchicine or Indocid. Two or three weeks after the acute attack has subsided the patient should take Allopurinol (Zyloric) or Probenecid (Benemid) to lower the uric acid in the blood. These two drugs should not be taken during the acute attack or just after an attack of gout as they may bring on the attack again. Patients should also avoid taking offal and wines.

Renal Complications of Gout

In patients with gout, renal disease is the most common and serious complication. There are two types of renal involvement in gout:

1. *Kidney Stones*

Patients with gout may pass 3 types of stones: uric acid stones, calcium oxalate stones and mixed urate-calcium stones.

Uric acid stones are formed in the presence of acidic urine which contains plenty of uric acid. These stones are easy to treat and prevent. The patient should drink enough water to produce 3 litres of urine daily. In addition, he has to take sodium bicarbonate solution to make the urine alkaline as uric acid stones form in an acidic urine. So if the urine is alkaline, stones are less likely to form. Allopurinol can also be prescribed to lower the uric acid level in the blood and urine.

Calcium oxalate stones are more commonly formed in patients with gout than in the normal population. This is because uric acid in the urine forms a nidus for the deposition and growth of calcium oxalate crystals.

2. *Gouty* Nephropathy

Passage of protein in the urine is the first clinical sign. Sometimes there may be pus cells or blood in the urine if the patient also has kidney stones and urine infection. With time, "very rarely" some patients with gouty nephropathy may slowly develop mild renal impairment. Histologically there is microtophi and chronic interstitial inflammation in the kidney. Several investigators question the existence of specific gouty nephropathy as a primary event in patients with clinical gout. This is because these patients often have hypertension, diabetes mellitus or hyperlipemia, all of which can cause nephrosclerosis with accompanying azotemia. Treatment consists of liberal intake of fluid, with avoidance of offal and wines. Allopurinol should also be prescribed as it will reduce the formation of uric acid and may arrest the renal deterioration.

DIETARY FACTORS AND CALCIUM NEPHROLITHIASIS[1]

1. Upper urinary tract stones correlate with economic affluence (high protein diet).
2. Bladder stones in Southern Asia and India — related to protein malnutrition,
3. Vegetarianism protects against stones though increases urinary oxalate excretion.
4. Protein load increases urinary calcium, oxalate and uric acid.

High Level of Dietary Protein

1. Population studies — high consumption of animal protein increases prevalence of upper tract stones.
2. High dietary protein increases urinary calcium, uric acid and oxalate. High intake of animal protein increases endogenous production of oxalate.
3. Dietary protein restriction has citraturic and hypocalciuric effect.
4. Low incidence of stones in vegetarians.
5. Prophylactic effect of dietary protein reduction in hypercalciurics, hyperuricosurics.

Other Factors

1. Increase in dietary **sodium** causes inhibition of Ca^{++} and Na^+ reabsorption at proximal tubule and loop of Henle.
2. Increased ingestion of **oxalate** in diet (spinach, rhubarb, peanuts, strawberries, chocolates, tea) causes recurrent stones.
3. Dietary **calcium** restriction is detrimental because negative Ca^{++} balance leads to bone reabsorption. It also causes secondary hyperoxaluria.
4. **Fluid** therapy is good. But no carbohydrate or oxalate (fruit juice) should be taken or benefit will be negated by increased excretion of lithogenic components.

Dietary Therapy

1. Patients whose dietary Na^+, protein, oxalate and calcium are excessive, OR urinary volume low, require dietary modification.
2. Reduce: <100 mEq/day Na^+, 1 gm/kg protein, 1000–1500 mg Ca^{++}, avoid oxalate-rich food, at least 3 litres urine per day.
3. High dietary fibre lowers dietary Ca^{++} and oxalate absorption.
4. Assess: 24-hour urinary Na^+ excretion, 24-hour urinary urea excretion (protein intake), 24-hour urine volume (fluid intake).

REFERENCE

1. Kidney Int. 1988, **34**:544–555.

CHAPTER 13

Diabetes Mellitus and the Kidney

The Nephrology of Diabetes Mellitus (DM) embraces a broad spectrum of clinical renal entities ranging from diabetic nephropathy, urinary tract infections, papillary necrosis to autonomic bladder with all its complications. Diabetic Nephropathy (DiabNx) however, is by far the predominant clinical entity accounting for more than 90% of the renal problems associated with DM. This chapter focuses on the treatment of DiabNx which is the commonest cause of end stage renal failure (ESRF) in Singapore accounting for 40% of new end stage renal failure seen every year.[1] In the USA, DiabNx is the commonest cause of ESRF (40%), Sweden 20% and Australia 12%. The trend for increasing incidence of DM should be a cause for concern for everyone. Previously chronic glomerulonephritis used to be the leading cause in Singapore.

DiabNx rarely develops before 10 years duration of DM. About 30% to 40% of patients with Type I and II DM will develop DiabNx but those patients who survive 35 years of DM without developing DiabNx are at extremely low risk of doing so in future.[2] In the last decade several interventional strategies have resulted in slowing the decline of renal function and the 10 year mortality rate of patients with DiabNx has been reduced from 70% to 20%.[3] Therapeutic strategies in DiabNx nowadays include strict glycemic control, strict control of hypertension, use of angiotensin converting enzyme (ACE) inhibitors or ATRA, dietary protein restriction and control of hypercholesterolaemia.

Natural History of Diabetic Nephropathy

There are 5 stages in the natural history. Stage I: Here there is glomerular hyperfiltration and renal enlargement. Albuminuria may be present. Stage II: Normoalbuminuria. With control of hyperglycemia, microalbuminuria disappears. Stage III: Incipient Diabetic Nephropathy. After 5 to 7 years, especially in patients where blood sugar is not well controlled, microalbuminuria appears again. If blood sugar is well controlled again, microalbuminuria may disappear. Stage IV: Overt or Established Diabetic Nephropathy. There is now persistent macroalbuminuria (dipstix for protein is positive, total urinary protein excretion more than 150 mg/day). Overt Diabetic Nephropathy is no longer reversible. With time there is accompanying decline in GFR with rise in blood pressure. Stage V: End Stage Renal Failure.

I. Role of Glycemic Control in Diabetic Nephropathy

Poor glycemic control initiates complications of DM and once established DiabNx progresses inexorably. Metabolic control of DM is important for progression of DiabNx. Even if the blood pressure is controlled the impact of metabolic control of blood sugar is still obvious.[4] In the recent Diabetic Control and Complications Trial (DCCT)[5] from the DCCT Research Group, American Diabetes Research Association, 1993, a total of 1441 patients with IDDM (726 with no retinopathy and 715 with retinopathy) were randomly assigned to either (i) Intensive therapy with insulin pump or 3 or more times a day injections or (ii) conventional therapy on once or twice daily insulin injections. The goal was pre-parandial blood glucose of 3.9 to 6.7 mmol/litre, post-parandial blood glucose less than 10 mmol/litre and HbA1C less than 6.05%. The mean duration of follow up was 6.5 years.

The conclusions were that strict glycemic control (i) in normoalbuminuric diabetics delays onset and slows progression of DiabNx (ii) in incipient DiabNx, it retards progression of nephropathy and (iii) in overt DiabNx, there were no beneficial effects in retardation of renal disease.

Therefore strict glycemic control in DiabNx is important for patients with normoalbuminuria and microalbuminuria (incipient DiabNx). Their HbA1C should be less than 7% but in those with overt or established DiabNx, that is, presence of macroalbuminuria (positive test for protein on dipstix) one should beware of hypoglycemia as renal failure progresses as insulin is metabolized by the proximal tubules of the kidney and the half life of insulin is prolonged as renal failure progresses. Blood glucose should be monitored regularly and insulin or oral hypoglycemics reduced accordingly.

II. Role of Hypertension in Diabetic Nephropathy

Hypertension aggravates underlying renal disease irrespective of the type of renal disease. Aggravation of the underlying renal disease itself also causes both hypertension and deterioration of renal function. In DiabNx, prospective studies have shown preservation of renal function by anti-hypertensive therapy. Mogensen in 1976[6] showed that improved blood pressure control in patients with DiabNx led to dramatic slowing on the rate of decline of the renal function. Hypertension is therefore a most important risk factor in DiabNx. In patients where the mean arterial blood pressure (MAP) is significantly reduced there is significant decrease in the rate of decline of the GFR. There is also a significant decrease in the rate of urinary albumin excretion. In a patient with DiabNx the optimum BP should be less than 140/90.

In the choice of an anti-hypertensive agent one should consider the metabolic and reno-protective effect. Thiazides and beta-blockers adversely affect glucose tolerance and lipid profile though they decrease proteinuria; whereas ACE Inhibitors, ATRA and calcium channel blockers decrease proteinuria without these adverse effects. In patients with DiabNx there is glomerular hyperfiltration where there is angiotensin II mediated vasoconstriction of the efferent glomerular arteriole. ACE Inhibitors cause efferent arteriolar vasodilatation at the glomerulus thereby decreasing intra-glomerular hypertension and reducing proteinuria.

III. Role of Angiotensinogen Converting Enzyme Inhibitors

As early as 1934, Cambier[7] had already shown that GFR was increased in patients with DiabNx. Before insulin therapy, GFR was 40% above normal and with treatment there was a reduction to 25% above normal. The increase in GFR was related to glycemic control. Morgensen in 1976[6] demonstrated that patients with the highest GFR were those destined to develop overt DiabNx. Patients with DiabNx have activated renin-angiotensin system making ACE Inhibitors effective in influencing renal hemodynamics. Aurell in 1992[7] showed that captopril therapy (25 mg thrice daily) reduced the rate of decline of GFR by 50%. ACE Inhibitor also has reno-protective effect. Enalapril, a long acting ACE Inhibitor has anti-proteinuric effect compared to metoprolol.

In 1993, Lewis et al[8] published the results of a collaborative study to determine if captopril, an ACE Inhibitor has reno-protective effects. It was a multicentre, randomised, double blind controlled trial with 207 patients on captopril and 202 patients on placebo. The primary study end point was a doubling of baseline creatinine to at least 2.0 mg/dl and the secondary analyses included the length of time to the combined end point of death, dialysis, transplantation and changes in renal function assessed in terms of serum creatinine concentration, 24 hour creatinine clearance and urinary protein excretion. The median follow up period was 3 years.

The results of the study showed that there were less patients in the captopril group who doubled their serum creatinine (n = 25) compared to 43 in the placebo group (p < 0.007). The mean rate of decline in creatinine clearance (11+/−21 ml/min) of the captopril group was slower than 17+/−21 ml/min in the placebo group (p < 0.03).

In the captopril group there was a 50% reduction in risk of death, dialysis and transplantation independent of the small disparity in BP between the 2 groups. The conclusion of the study was that captopril protects against deterioration in renal function in IDDM patients with nephropathy and is significantly more effective than BP control alone. The reno-protective effects were independent of its effect on BP. ACE Inhibitor therapy therefore should be recommended to diabetic patients with incipient DiabNx (presence of microalbuminuria) and those with overt or established DiabNx (dipstix positive or presence of macroalbuminuria).

However, there are certain precautions during use of ACE Inhibitor therapy. ACE Inhibitor is contraindicated in patients with renal artery stenosis and should be used with caution in patients with renal impairment as the drop in intraglomerular BP due to efferent arteriolar vasodilatation will cause further lowering of the GFR leading to further worsening of existing renal impairment. Since ACE Inhibitor is anti-aldosterone and anti-angiotensin it will cause retention of K+, giving rise to hyperkalaemia and salt and water depletion as it counters the physiological functions of aldosterone and angiotensin to retain salt and water.

IV. RENAAL Trial

Recently[16] in a randomized multicentre control trial, RENAAL (Reduction of End points in NIDDM with Angiotensin II Receptor Antagonist, Losartan), involving 1513 patients from 29 countries with NIDDM of which 751 patients in the treatment group were on Losartan 50 mg to 100 mg daily compared to 762 patients given placebo, both groups also continuing treatment for hypertension with conventional BP medicine, excluding ACE inhibitors and other Angiotensin Receptor Blocker (ATRA) there was a 28% reduction in development of End Stage Renal Disease among the patients treated with Losartan. Proteinuria in the Losartan treated group decreased by 35% compared to those on placebo. The trial was conducted over a 3 and a half years period.

V. The Role of Dietary Protein Restriction in DiabNx

In 1981, Brenner[9] demonstrated that increased dietary protein accentuated the decline in renal function of one and two-thirds nephrectomised rats. Walker[10] in 1989 showed that protein restriction on the other hand could retard the progression of renal failure in patients with renal failure. Zeller in 1991[11] reported that dietary protein restriction slowed the rate of decline of GFR in IDDM patients (3 ml/min compared to 12 ml/min in controls).

Our current practice for patients with DiabNx is to recommend a 0.8 gm/Kg BW protein diet. A 50 kg weight patient will be prescribed a 40 gm protein diet. The American Diabetic Association recommends a 0.6 gm/Kg BW protein diet but such zealous dieting only leads to malnutrition by the time the patient requires dialysis. We would advise the patient to stop dieting when serum creatinine is about 500 micromol/litre to avoid the dangers of malnutrition.

VI. The Role of Hyperlipidemia in Diabetic Nephropathy

Hyperlipidemia is an important factor accelerating loss of kidney function in renal disease. In patients with any form of renal disease, hyperlipidemia is a significant risk factor. As early as 1967, French[12] and later Kasiske in 1970[13] demonstrated that the experimental rat model developed accelerated glomerulosclerosis when fed a high cholesterol diet. Mulec in 1990[14] showed that patients with DiabNx with serum cholesterol less than 7.0 mmol/litre had a slower decline of GFR (2.3 ml/min) compared to those with serum cholesterol more than 7 mmol/litre (GFR 8.4 ml/min) (p < 0.01).

Control of serum lipids is important, especially LDL-cholesterol. Oxidised LDL-cholesterol causes mesangial cell proliferation at a low dose and is cytotoxic at a high dose[15]. Lipoprotein also binds to GBM altering its filtration property adversely leading to proteinuria. One should aim to decrease LDL-cholesterol to less than 3 to 4 mmol/litre. Treatment for hypercholesterolaemia includes dietary control as well as cholesterol lowering drugs.

VII. Indications for Referral of a Patient with Diabetes Mellitus to a Nephrologist

The question of when to refer the patient to a nephrologist has often been asked.

1. Ideally, the patient should be referred when there is microalbuminuria (albumin excretion rate more 30 mg/ day but less than 150 mg/day). At this stage the patient already has incipient diabetic nephropathy which may still be reversible.

2. When the patient has proteinuria on dipstix (macroalbuminuria or proteinuria more than 150 mg/ day) or when the patient has the nephrotic syndrome he should be referred. At this stage it means that the patient already has overt or established diabetic nephropathy.

3. A patient with microscopic haematuria or other urinary abnormality (pyuria) needs referral as this may indicate that he has non diabetic nephropathy and such a patient should be referred to exclude other types of renal disease.

4. Presence of hypertension may indicate a patient with incipient or overt diabetic nephropathy.

5. Patients with renal impairment, indicating overt or established diabetic nephropathy.

IN CONCLUSION

For the patient with Diabetes Mellitus with no proteinuria (normoalbuminuria) intensive blood glucose control as well as cholesterol control is mandatory. For those with incipient diabetic nephropathy (microalbuminuria excretion rate more than 30 mg/day, but dipstix negative), intensive blood glucose control, control of hypertension, ACEI/ATRA therapy, dietary protein restriction and cholesterol control is necessary.

In patients with overt or established diabetic nephropathy one should monitor for decline in renal function and decrease the dose of insulin or oral hypoglycemics accordingly to prevent hypoglycemia. Control of hypertension, ACE Inhibitor therapy, dietary protein restriction and treatment of hypercholesterolaemia and hypertriglyceridemia is necessary. The goals in the management of a patient with Diabetes Mellitus is to prevent the development of Diabetic Nephropathy. If the patient already has overt or established Diabetic Nephropathy one should still attempt to retard the progression of renal disease to prevent renal failure.

REFERENCES

1. Woo KT: Renal Replacement Therapy in Singapore. In: Dialysis Therapy in the 1990s. Editor: H Tanaka. Contributions to Nephrology, Karger, Basel. 1990, **82**:6–14.

2. Breyer JA: Diabetic Nephropathy in Insulin Dependent patients. *Amer J Kid Disease*. 1992, **20**:533–547.

3. Parving HH, Hommel E: Prognosis in Diabetic Nephropathy. *Br Med J*. 1989, **299**:230–233.

4. Mogensen CE: Prevention and Treatment of Renal Disease in Insulin Dependent Diabetes Mellitus. *Semin Nephrol*. 1990, **10**:261–273.

5. The Diabetes Control and Complications Trial (DCCT) Research Group: The effect of intensive treatment of Diabetes on the development and progression of long term complications in Insulin Dependent Diabetes mellitus. *New Engl J Med*. 1993, **329**:977–986.

6. Mogensen CE : Progression of nephropathy in long term diabetics with proteinuria and effect of initial antihypertensive treatment. *Scand J Clin Lab Invest.* 1976, **36**:383–388.

7. Aurell M, Bjorck S: Determinants of progressive renal disease in diabetes mellitus. *Kid Int.* 1992, **41**:S38–S42.

8. Lewis EJ, Hunsicker LG, Bain RP, Rohde RD for the collaborative study group: The effect of angiotensin converting enzyme inhibition on Diabetic Nephropathy. *New Engl J Med.* 1993, **329**:456–462.

9. Brenner BM, Meyer TW, Hostetter TH: Dietary protein and the progressive nature of kidney disease. *New Engl J Med.* 1982, **307**:652–659.

10. Walker JD, Dodds R, Murrells TJ, Bending JJ, Keen H, Viberti GC: Restriction of dietary protein and progression of renal failure in diabetic nephropathy. Lancet. 1989, **2**:1411–1415.

11. Zeller K, Whittaker E, Sullivan L, Raskin P, Jacobson HR: Effect of restricting dietary protein on progression of renal failure in patients with insulin-dependent diabetes mellitus. *New Engl J Med.* 1991, **324**:78–84.

12. French JW, Yamanaka BS, Ostwald R: Dietary induced glomerulosclerosis in the guinea pig. *Arch Pathol.* 1967, **83**:204–220.

13. Kasiske BL, O'Donell MP, Schmitz PG, Kim Y: Renal injury of diet induced hypercholesterolaemia in rats. *Kid Int.* 1990, **37**:880–891.

14. Mulec H, Johnson SA, Bjorck S: Relation between serum cholesterol and diabetic nephropathy. *Lancet.* 1990, **335**:1537–1538.

15. Diamond JR, Karnovsky MJ: Focal and Segmental Glomerulosclerosis: Analogies to Atherosclerosis. *Kid Int.* 1988, **33**:917–924.

16. Brenner BM, Cooper ME, de Zeeuw D, Keanne WF, Mitch WE, Parving HH, Remuzgi G, Snapinn SM, Zhang ZX, Shahinfar S for the RENAAL Study Investigators: Effects of Losartan on Renal and cardiovascular outcome in patients with Type 2 Diabetes and Nephropathy. *N Engl J Med.* 2001, **345**(12):861–869.

CHAPTER 14

Fluid and Electrolytes

SODIUM AND WATER

1. Regulation of serum Na^+ concentration effected via thirst-neurohypophyseal-renal axis.
2. Osmolality of solution refers to concentration in solution of osmotically active solute.
   Serum Osmolality = (Na + K)2 + Glucose ÷ 18 + Urea ÷ 6
   Normal = 285 ± 5 m Osmol/l. If SI units used, not necessary to divide by 18 and 6.
3. Changes in serum osmolality will cause osmoreceptors to increase or decrease the release of ADH to conserve or excrete water.
4. SIADH: Normal control of ADH release is lost. Secretion of hormone is independent of body's needs to conserve water.

SODIUM (Na⁺)

Na^+ is the osmotic stuffing of the body. It has little metabolic activity per se. In contrast to K^+ which is an intracellular cation, Na^+ is an extracellular cation.

Distribution

Plasma 11%, interstitial lymph 30%, cartilage and connective tissue 12%, bone 42%, transcellular and intracellular 2.5% each.

Body Na^+: Bone 2 600 mEq, muscle 420 mEq, ECF 2 500 mEq, others 135 mEq.

Symptoms of Hyponatraemia

Lack of concentration, apathy, headache, anorexia, nausea, vomiting. In severe cases there will be fits and patients may be comatose. Reflexes are depressed and temperature may be subnormal.

Symptoms of Hypernatraemia

Irritability, confusion, hyper-reflexia, variable pyrexia and coma.

Hyponatraemia

1. Dilutional Hyponatraemia (Expansion of body fluids)
   i. Hysterical polydipsia
   ii. Inappropriate ADH (SIADH)
   iii. Renal failure
   iv. Cirrhosis
   v. Nephrotic Syndrome
   Treatment: Water restriction.

2. Absolute salt depletion (Contraction of body fluids)
   i. Gastrointestinal loss: Vomit, diarrhoea
   ii. Renal loss: Addison's disease, uraemia, recovery from acute tubular necrosis (ATN)
   Treatment: Hypertonic fluids (normal saline, 3% saline).

Hypernatraemia with Expansion of Body Fluids

Infusion of normal saline in excess will cause hypernatraernia with salt and water overload.

Treatment: Salt and water restriction; diuretic therapy.

Hypernatremia with Contraction of Body Fluids

1. Inadequate Water Intake (Patients in coma, palsy, hypothalamic lesions)
   i. Amount of water required conditioned by diet and concentration ability of kidneys.
   ii. Progressive hypernatraemia in unconscious patients fed high protein and high calorie diets through Ryle's tube.
   iii. Or I.V. infusion of aminoacids and hyperosmolar fluids.
   iv. Patients require more water for excretion of end products of metabolism. Provision of adequate supply of water is important.
   v. Treatment: Body fluid expansion with hyponatraemic infusions.

2. Renal Water Wasting
   Either due to:
   i. Diabetes insipidus (neurohypophyseal, nephrogenic).
   ii. OR: Intrinsic Renal Disease like Pyelonephritis, Medullary Disease, Advanced Glomerular Disease (renal impairment), Hypercalcaemia and Hypokalaemia.

3. Given normal thirst mechanism, polyuria rarely causes hypernatraemia because of polydipsia induced by the thirst.

4. However, if water intake is restricted or impaired consciousness, hypernatraemic contraction develops.

Oedema

1. Cardiac, hepatic and renal cause due to retention of salt and water resulting from hypoperfusion of kidney and increased ADH.
2. Excess infusion of saline.
3. Toxaemia of pregnancy due to intense Na^+ reabsorption and altered renal haemodynamics.
4. Idiopathic oedema of women. Oestrogens have been implicated as they promote Na^+ retention by renal tubules. Another theory postulates capillary leakage.
5. Mineralocorticoid excess. Aldosterone causes Na^+ and water retention.
6. Hypothyroidism due to myxoedema.
7. Diabetes mellitus due to capillary microangiopathy.
8. Chronic hypokalaemia increases tubular reabsorption of Na^+.
9. Drugs like oestrogens, vasodilators (diazoxide, hydrallazine, clonidine, lithium carbonate) cause Na^+ retention by renal tubule.
10. Arteriovenous fistula increases cardiac output and Na^+ retention.

Idiopathic (Cyclical) Oedema

1. Disorder of women where there is weight gain and oedema, often in obese females.
2. There is Na^+ and water retention in the upright position. Diuresis occurs with recumbency.
3. Exclude diabetes mellitus, hypothyroidism and premenstrual oedema.
4. Aetiology: Oestrogen, diuretic induced stimulation of the renin angiotensin aldosterone system, inability to decrease ADH, capillary leakiness, inability to increase natriuretic hormone.

5. Treatment: Stop diuretics, maximum weight gain is evident by 10 days of stopping diuretics, and spontaneous diuresis subsequently ensues. Sodium restriction may be required initially to control oedema formation.

Natriuretic Hormone (NH)

1. Saline expansion in dogs produces a brisk natriuresis because of humoral substance inhibiting Na^+ reabsorption at renal tubule (HE de Wardener).
2. In congestive heart failure, advanced cirrhosis and nephrotic syndrome, there is relentless Na^+ retention. This could be due to a lack of natriuretic hormone.
3. Natriuretic hormone may be the cause of certain forms of essential hypertension.
4. A Hypothalarnic Factor (HF) has been isolated which promotes Na^+ and water excretion in renal tubule but inhibits Na/K ATPase in other tissues (vasoconstriction).

Atrial Natriuretic Peptide (ANP)

1. A potent natriuretic and vasorelaxant 24-amino acid peptide found in granules of the heart's atria.
2. It does not inhibit Na/K ATPase. It causes greater natriuresis and diuresis.
3. Effects:
   i. Vasorelaxant on vascular smooth muscles.
   ii. Renal haemodynamics: ANP causes increased GFR, Na^+ and fluid excretion.
   iii. On BP: ANP causes a dose dependent reduction.
   iv. On the Renin-Angiotensin System: ANP is anti-Renin. It decreases its secretion and opposes vasoconstriction.
   v. On Aldosterone: ANP opposes its action and decreases Na^+ reiention.

Syndrome of Inappropriate Secretion of ADH

1. Normal control of ADH release is lost. The hormone is secreted independently of the body's needs to conserve water.
2. Urine is concentrated and water retention occurs.
3. There is expansion of body fluids and circulating blood volume.
4. This is accompanied by increased renal perfusion and GFR with decreased Na^+ reabsorption as Aldosterone production is shut off.
5. Hyponatraemia is a consequence of water retention and Na^+ wastage.
6. With time, a new steady state develops where intake and excretion of water and Na^+ are in balance; but serum Na^+ is now set at a new level.
7. In a patient with hyponatraemia and normal rate of Na^+ excretion, SIADH should be suspected. In other words, the patient is in Na^+ balance when Urinary Output = Intake of Na^+.
8. If sodium is infused, sodium diuresis will result with no change in serum Na^+.

Causes of SIADH

I. By the neurohypophysis,
    1. CNS disorders: Head injury, meningitis, encephalitis, brain tumour and subarachnoid haemorrhage.
    2. Lung disorders: TB, pneumonia.
    3. Endocrine diseases: Addison's disease, myxoedema and hypopituitarism.

II. By tumours
    Cancer of the lungs, duodenum and pancreas. Thymoma.

Treatment of Salt Loss

1. Infuse normal saline or 3% saline. Sometimes salt tablets may be sufficient. Free salt diet.
2. Measure 24-hour urinary excretion of Na^+ to determine urinary salt loss.
3. 1 gm oral NaCl = 17 mEq of Na^+, 1 litre of normal saline = 154 mEq, 1 litre of 3% saline = 513 mEq of Na^+.

Calculation of Sodium Deficit

If Body Weight is 65 kg and serum Na^+ 120 mEq/l,
Na^+ deficit = 140 − 120 = 20 mEq/l
Body Water = 60% of Body Weight

$$\text{Hence } Na^+ \text{ deficit} = \frac{65 \times 60 \times 20}{100} = 780 \text{ mEq/l}$$

$$= 5 \text{ litres } 0.9\% \text{ NaCl}$$

Give 1/2 the calculated Na^+ deficit in 12–24 hours. Check serum Na^+ the next day and using same calculation see how much more Na^+ is needed.

POTASSIUM

1. Body K^+ Distribution:

   Plasma — 0.4%
   Interstitial Lymph — 1.0%
   Dense Connective Tissue and Cartilage — 0.4%
   Bone — 7.6%
   Intracellular — 89.6%
   Transcellular — 1.0%
   Note that most of the K^+ stays intracellularly in contrast to Na^+ which is mainly extracellular.

2. Total Body K^+ (TBK^+)

   — measured by K^{42} or K^{40}
   Muscle cells — 3 000 mEq
   Extracellular fluid — 65 mEq
   Liver — 200 mEq
   RBC — 235 mEq
   Urine — 92 mEq/day
   Stool — 8 mEq/day

3. K^+ is excreted in the urine via the distal tubule at a rate proportional to the reabsorption of Na^+.

4. In Acidosis, H^+ goes into the cell and K^+ comes out of the cell. Hence serum K^+ becomes high (Hyperkalaemia).

5. In Alkalosis, K^+ stays in the cell; so serum K^+ is low (Hypokalaemia). H^+ comes out of the cell to compensate.

6. K^+ is responsible for Enzyme Action in the cell. Conduction of nerve and muscle impulses (transmembrane potential difference) requires K^+.

K^+ Depletion

1. Increased loss in urine
   i. In Hyperaldosteronism, Na^+ is retained while K^+ is lost into the urine.
   ii. Cortisol excess (Cushing's) too causes retention of Na^+ and loss of K^+ giving rise to Hypokalaemic Alkalosis.
   iii. Diuretics (Frusemide, Chlorothiazide) cause loss of Na^+ and K^+ into the urine, resulting in Hypokalaemic Alkalosis.
   iv. Renal Tubular Acidosis is associated with K^+ loss in the urine since the excretion of H^+ into the urine is impaired.

    v. Alkalosis is associated with K^+ loss in the urine.

    vi. Bartter's syndrome where there is hyper-renin hyperaldosteronism resulting in hypokalaemia.

2. Loss in gastrointestinal tract

    — Vomiting, diarrhoea, Ryle's tube aspiration and fistulae all result in K^+ loss.

3. Decreased intake

    Patients who are starved have low K^+ due to decreased intake.

Effects of K^+ Depletion

K^+ depletion may cause:

1. Hypokalaemia.
2. Renal Tubular Necrosis with Nephrogenic Diabetes Insipidus.
3. Treatment: Administer KCl. Never give KCl intravenously in a bolus dose for it will kill the patient. Intravenous K^+ must be given gradually by I.V. drip infusion slowly over 1 hour, if necessary under ECG monitoring. Give oral KCl if patient can take orally and urgent correction is not necessary. 1 gm KCl = 13.3 mEq/l.

Hyperkalaemia

Causes:

1. Fever, trauma and infection will cause cell damage with release of K^+.
2. Any catabolic or hypercatabolic states; conditions associated with acidosis except in states where there is urinary loss of K^+ (renal tubular acidosis, ureterosigmoidostomy, ileo-conduit).
3. Renal failure is a very common cause.

Treatment of Hyperkalaemia

1. Stop all sources of K^+ (fruits and juices).
2. Administer I.V. calcium gluconate or calcium chloride (10 ml slowly) to combat the effects of hyperkalaemia on the heart.
3. Give I.V. insulin 12 units together with 50 ml of 50% dextrose either as a bolus dose or over 1 hour in a drip.
4. I.V. $NaHCO_3$ 8.4% (10 ml) to combat acidosis which is often present.
5. Commence Oral Resonium A 15 gm 6 hourly if patient can take orally. If patient cannot take orally, give Resonium Retention Enema, 30 gm 8 hourly instead.
6. Check the serum electrolytes and repeat bolus doses of insulin and dextrose 4 hourly.
7. If hyperkalaemia persists, dialysis would have to be considered.
8. Treat the cause of hyperkalaemia wherever possible.

Effects of Hyperkalaemia

1. Early phase: No signs are present.
2. Late Phase: Flaccid palsy, shallow respiration, anxiety, anaesthetic.
   ECG: Tented T, ST depressed, Bradycardia, Prolong PR, Prolong QRS, Nodal Rhythm, Ventricular Arrhythmias, Cardiac Arrest in Dilatation.

MAGNESIUM

Total Body Mg = 2 400 mEq
Bone contains 2/3, soft tissue 1/3 and ECF 1%.

Function

1. Enzymes require it for their function.
2. Stabilisation of membrane potential.
3. Permissive action for Parathyroid Hormone.

Mg Deficiency

1. Fatigue, lethargy, weakness, tremors, fits, arrhythmia, paresthesia, psychosis, Chovstek and Trousseau's sign.
2. May be associated with Hypo Ca^{++}, Hypo K^+, Hypo Na^+.
3. Causes: Diarrhoea, alcohol, diuretics, aldosteronism, hypoparathyroidism.
4. Treat with $MgCl_2$ (40–50 mEq/day).
   1 gm $MgSO_4$ $7H_2O$ = 8.13 mEq/l Magnesium
   1 gm $MgCl_2$ $6H_2O$ = 9.15 mEq/l Magnesium

Hypermagnesaemia: Associated with hyporeflexia, coma and cardiac arrest.

CHAPTER 15

Acid-Base Balance

PATHOGENESIS OF METABOLIC ACIDOSIS

Non-carbonic acid-base equilibrium in the ECF compartment of the body is modulated by 3 processes: (1) cellular metabolism, (2) intestinal absorption and secretion, and (3) renal acidification.

The net renal input of bicarbonate into the ECF and the net endogenous acid production are approximately equal, so that the plasma bicarbonate and blood pH are kept constant.

NET ENDOGENOUS ACID PRODUCTION

Net endogenous acid production increases because of:
1. Disordered cellular metabolic processes, eg. ketoacidosis, hypoxia (lactic acidosis).
2. Loading of the normal metabolic pathway with ingested noncarbonic precursors, eg. ammonium chloride.
3. External losses of abnormally large amounts of gastrointestinal secretions containing bicarbonate, eg. diarrhoea; external drainage of pancreatic, biliary or small bowel secretions; ureterosigmoidostomy; ingestion of calcium chloride, magnesium sulphate, cholestyramine.

PHYSIOLOGICAL RESPONSE TO METABOLIC ACIDOSIS OF EXTERNAL ORIGIN

1. In the Pulmonary Response to metabolic acidosis, the CO_2 tension of body fluid decreases and as a consequence the concentrations of carbonic acid and H^+, which are in equilibrium with CO_2 decreases concomitantly.
2. In the Renal Response, the net renal input of bicarbonate into the ECF of the body increases.
3. With increasing degrees of acidosis (low plasma bicarbonate), hyperventilation increases, but this is insufficient to prevent lowering of blood pH.
4. Hence respiratory compensation offers little protection in severe metabolic acidosis.

RENAL RESPONSE TO METABOLIC ACIDOSIS OF EXTRARENAL ORIGIN

1. When endogenous acid production becomes great, the amount of bicarbonate delivered to the ECF by the kidneys (via renal venous blood) begins to exceed the amount delivered to the kidneys (in renal artery) by a greater amount than normal (ie. 1.0 mEq/kg body weight per day).
2. If the rate of endogenous acid production remains abnormal for several days, net renal input of bicarbonate progressively increases till it becomes adequate.
3. In persisting metabolic acidosis, bone supplies additional base.
4. The kidney's ability to correct metabolic acidosis depends on excretion of buffered H^+ (Titratable Acid and NH_4^+)

CONSEQUENCES OF METABOLIC ACIDOSIS

1. Acidosis leads to circulatory collapse.
2. Decreases cardiac response to catecholamines.

3. Depresses myocardial contractile force.
4. Increases pulmonary arteriolar resistance.
5. Venous constriction causes redistribution of large amounts of blood into the central circulation, leading to heart failure.
6. Circulatory insufficiency leads to tissue hypoxia and increased lactic production.
7. Movement of potassium out of somatic muscle cells causes hyperkalaemia.

CAUSES OF METABOLIC ACIDOSIS

I. Hyperchloraemic, Normal Anion Gap Acidosis

1. Acid load: Ammonium chloride, hyperalimentation.
2. Bicarbonate losses: diarrhoea, fistulae, ureterosigmoidostomy.
3. Defects in urinary acidification: Proximal renal tubular acidosis, distal renal tubular acidosis.
4. Renal impairment.

II. Normochloraemic, High Anion Gap Acidosis

1. Causes: Lactic acidosis; diabetic, alcoholic and starvation acidosis; drug and toxin induced acidosis; advanced uraemic acidosis.
2. Addition to body of non-chloride acid load will cause high anion gap acidosis.
3. Anion gap = $Na^+ - (Cl^- + HCO_3^-)$.
   Normally this is about 12 mEq/l (range: 8 to 16 mEq/l).
4. In practice: $(Na^+ + K^+) - (Cl^- + HCO_3) \geq 20$ (abnormal).
5. Occurs if anion does not undergo glomerular filtration (uraemic acid anions) OR anion filtered but readily absorbed (ketoacids, lactate).

LACTIC ACIDOSIS (COHEN AND WOODS)

1. Lactic acid in blood causes decreased bicarbonate and elevation in lactate concentration and anion gap.
2. Considered abnormal if blood lactate > 4 mEq/l (normal is 1 mEq/l).

   Type A: Poor tissue perfusion,

   i. Shock (cardiogenic, haemorrhagic, septic),

   ii. Acute hypoxaemia,

   iii. Carbon monoxide poisoning

   Type B:

   i. Common diseases like diabetes mellitus, renal failure, liver disease, infection.

   ii. Drugs, toxins like phenformin, metformin, ethanol methanol, salicylates.

   iii. Hereditary disorders like pyruvate dehydrogenase deficiency, methylmalonic aciduria.

SYMPTOMS OF LACTIC ACIDOSIS

Hyperventilation, abdominal pain, disturbed consciousness, inadequate cardiopulmonary function (Type A), leukocytosis, hypoglycaemia, hyperkalaemia.

TREATMENT OF LACTIC ACIDOSIS

1. Treat underlying cause.
2. Vasodilator nitroprusside improves hypoperfusion by enhancing cardiac output, liver and renal blood flow. This will augment lactate removal.
3. Alkali therapy advocated if blood pH < 7.1. Danger of fluid overload because of large amounts of bicarbonate required.

4. Diuretics, ultrafiltration and bicarbonate haemodialysis can be used to remove lactic acid.
5. In treating acidosis, "overshoot alkalosis" may occur because of lactate conversion to bicarbonate by the liver, renal generation of bicarbonate and bicarbonate load from therapy.

TREATMENT OF METABOLIC ACIDOSIS

1. Mitigate severity of acidaemia and/or hyperkalaemia by reversal of pathogenetic processes. Give $NaHCO_3$.
   Correct if serum bicarbonate less than 15 mEq/l
   eg. if Serum Bicarbonate = 10 mEq/l
   $\frac{1}{3}$ Body Weight × Bicarbonate Deficit = x ml 8.4% $NaHCO_3$,
   $\quad \frac{1}{3}$ 60 kg × (25 − 10) = 20 × 15 = 300 ml 8.4% $NaHCO_3$.
2. Prevent recurrence of acidaemia by maintenance therapy.
3. It is not necessary to correct acidosis completely within minutes or hours as hyperventilation continues for hours after correction of acidaemia.
4. Rapid normalisation of plasma bicarbonate concentration is associated with inappropriate increase in arterial blood pH with occurrence of respiratory alkalosis.
5. Hypokalaemia is a complication of bicarbonate treatment. If serum K^+ is less than 4 mEq/l give KCl.

METABOLIC ALKALOSIS

The pH of blood is given by ratio of the bicarbonate concentration to dissolved CO_2 :

$$pH = 6.1 + \log \frac{HCO_3^-}{CO_2}$$

1. Plasma CO_2 tension maintained within very narrow limits through regulated excretion of CO_2 by lungs.
2. Kidney stabilises the concentration of serum bicarbonate.

Under certain circumstances, the kidney far exceeds its homeostatic responsibility. It operates to sustain a high serum bicarbonate concentration by:

1. **Generating Alkalosis:** Large amounts of $NaHCO_3$ are added to the blood.
2. The kidney's **capacity to reabsorb** $NaHCO_3$ may be greatly **augmented,** so that new $NaHCO_3$ whether generated by renal or extra-renal factors, is not lost into the urine.

SYMPTOMS OF METABOLIC ALKALOSIS

1. Like hypocalcaemia.
2. Mental confusion, obtundation, seizures, paraesthesia, cramps, tetany, arrhythmias.
3. Hypokalaemia is often an associated feature.

CAUSES OF METABOLIC ALKALOSIS

1. Exogenous bicarbonate loads like acute alkali administration, milk alkali syndrome.
2. Gastrointestinal origin: Vomiting, gastric aspiration, villous adenoma.
3. Renal origin: Diuretics, potassium depletion, Bartter's syndrome.
4. Mineralocorticoids: Primary aldosteronism, Cushing's syndrome, liquorice ingestion.

PATHOGENESIS OF METABOLIC ALKALOSIS

1. Bicarbonate Generation
   i. Renal: Excretion of NH_4^+ plus titratable acidity must exceed that required to neutralise acid load (dietary, metabolic acid production, alkaline faecal loss).
   ii. Dietary NaCl furnishes Na^+ which is returned to the blood as $NaHCO_3$; the anion Cl^- is excreted into urine as NH_4 Cl.
   iii. Extra-Renal: Acid loss due to vomiting; or alkaline gain, eg. milk-alkaline syndrome.
2. Maintenance of Metabolic Alkalosis
   Capacity of the kidney to reclaim bicarbonate must be enhanced by a rise in tubular reabsorption commensurate with the filtered load, ie. **augmentation** in capacity of kidney to reclaim filtered bicarbonate.

GENERATION OF METABOLIC ALKALOSIS

1. Three features are usually present before this can occur:
   i. Relatively high distal delivery of Na^+ salts.
   ii. Persistent mineralocorticoid excess.
   iii. K^+ deficiency occurring simultaneously.
2. Enhanced bicarbonate reclamation is also necessary.
3. Na^+ reabsorption results in H^+ secretion, urine pH falls, buffers are titrated; NH_3 diffuses into acid urine and is trapped as NH_4^+. For every mole of Na^+ reabsorbed, one mole of bicarbonate is reclaimed and this represents $NaHCO_3$ regeneration.
4. Giving diuretics to oedematous patient may result in increased Na^+ delivery distally. The resulting bicarbonate generation allows an increased capacity for bicarbonate reclamation.
5. Vomiting leads to loss of HCl associated with K^+ deficiency. The extra-renal generation of bicarbonate may be reclaimed by virtue of increased H^+ secretion in the proximal tubule.

MAINTENANCE OF METABOLIC ALKALOSIS

1. In situations where there is increased "proximal" bicarbonate reabsorption because of increasing H^+ secretion, eg. as in patients with K^+ deficiency. Though expansion of volume can override the effect of K^+ deficiency, if K^+ depletion is severe, it will still maintain alkalosis.
2. K^+ deficiency also augments "distal" H^+ secretion. In K^+ depletion, Na^+ is preferentially exchanged for H^+. This serves to reclaim bicarbonate.
3. Shrinkage in effective arterial blood volume causes a reduction in back-leak of bicarbonate into the proximal tubular lumen; thereby enhancing bicarbonate reclamation.
4. Mineralocorticoids (aldosterone) stimulate Na^+/H^+ process in cortical collecting tubule. This augments bicarbonate reclamation in the distal tubule. A necessary condition is K^+ deficiency.
5. In Summary: Bicarbonate reclamation is increased by contraction of Effective Arterial Blood Volume, K^+ deficiency and excess aldosterone.

TREATMENT OF METABOLIC ALKALOSIS

1. Remove stimulus to bicarbonate generation (excess mineralocorticoid, intragastric suck, diuretics).
2. Remove factors maintaining bicarbonate reabsorption like extracellular volume (ECV) contraction, low K^+.
3. For "saline responsive alkalosis" like those due to vomiting, nasogastric suction, diuretics, K^+ deficiency, alkalosis following bicarbonate therapy for organic acidosis, post hypercapnia alkalosis (because of high aldosterone), NaCl infusion and KCl replacement are usually sufficient.
4. In "saline resistant alkalosis" like Bartter's, Conn's, Cushing's and renal artery stenosis (RAS), magnesium deficiency and severe K^+ deficiency, saline infusion is of

no use. Treatment is aimed at the underlying cause. In RAS, alkalosis is due to non-oedematous aldosteronism (high aldosterone, low ECV).

5. For severe cases of alkalosis, titrate plasma bicarbonate with arginine HCl, NH_4 Cl or dilute HCl and increase bicarbonate excretion with acetazolamide.

THE ROLE OF CHLORIDE DEFICIENCY IN METABOLIC ALKALOSIS

1. NaCl and $NaHCO_3$ are the only two salts whose reabsorption is readily regulated by the kidney that can function to maintain the extracellular volume.
2. The extracellular volume will contract with chloride (Cl^-) restriction, unless alkalosis is produced by giving $NaHCO_3$
3. The role of Cl^- in metabolic alkalosis is due to its capacity to permit expansion or contraction of EC volume.
4. Cl^- restriction reduces EC volume, stimulates Na^+ retention and aldosterone secretion. The urine is free of Cl^- as the kidneys retain all filtered Na^+ salts, with Cl^- and bicarbonate reabsorbed.
5. If metabolic alkalosis is produced by extra-renal means, eg. gastric aspirate, the contraction of effective EC volume will maintain it.
6. Giving NaCl restores EC volume and relieves stimulus to Na^+ retention, Cl^- and bicarbonate are delivered distally and excreted in the urine and this corrects the alkalosis. The volume expanding effect of NaCl overcomes the effect of K^+ deficiency.

BARTTER'S SYNDROME

1. Metabolic alkalosis with hypokalaemia, juxta-glomerular apparatus (JGA) hyperplasia, hyper-renin hyperaldosteronism.

2. These patients have no oedema. They are normotensive, have elevated serum prostaglandins and prostacycline, polycythaemia, hypercalciuria and normal GFR.

3. In the differential diagnosis, consider vomiting, diuretics and laxatives. These conditions are associated with low urinary chloride and saline responsive alkalosis whereas Bartter's syndrome is associated with high urinary chloride and saline resistant alkalosis.

4. The underlying causation may be a defect in the reabsorption of NaCl at the ascending limb of Henle. This leads to ECV contraction which causes raised renin and aldosterone, which in turn causes alkalosis and hypokalaemia.

5. Prostaglandins have been found to inhibit NaCl reabsorption by the cortical ascending limb of Henle; hence the use of indocid, a prostaglandin synthetase inhibitor in the treatment of Bartter's syndrome.

6. Treatment: Potassium replacement, inhibition of renin-angiotensin aldosterone and prostaglandin systems using captopril and indocid. These measures are still empirical.

CHAPTER 16

Clinical Problems on Fluids, Electrolytes and Acid-Base Balance

Question 1

A 53 year-old-man presents with a duodenal ulcer, bronchopneumonia and diabetes mellitus.

Serum	Glucose	238	mg/dl	(13.2 mmol/l)
	Urea	360	mg/dl	(60 mmol/l)
	Creatinine	5.9	mg/dl	(522 μmol/l)
	Na	157	mmol/l	
	K	2.3	mmol/L	
	Cl	116	mmol/L	

Arterial	pH	7.5	
	Base Excess	10.2	
	SBC	34	mmol/L
	Oxygen Sat	95.9	%

1. Why is he hypernatraemic?
2. Calculate serum osmolality.
3. What is the acid-base disturbance?
4. Treatment.

Question 2
A 23-year-old woman presents with severe diarrhoea and laboured respiration. Her body weight is 65 kg.

Serum	Na	120	mmol/l	
	K	5.5	mmol/l	
	Cl	86	mmol/l	
	Urea	184	mg/dl	(30.7 mmol/l)
	Creatinine	5.1	mg/dl	(451 μmol/l)
	SBC	10	mmol/l	

Arterial   pH   7.21

1. What is the acid-base and electrolyte disorder?
2. Why are serum creatinine and urea raised?
3. Calculate sodium deficit.
4. Calculate bicarbonate deficit.

Question 3
A 43-year-old female has an ileal conduit because of tuberculous cystitis. Her body weight is 60 kg.

Serum	Na	137	mmol/l
	K	2.9	mmol/l
	Cl	115	mmol/l
	SBC	15	mmol/l

Arterial   pH   7.124

1. What is the acid-base disorder?
2. Explain hypokalaemia in this condition.
3. Calculate bicarbonate deficit.
4. What are long-term complications?

Question 4

A 13-year-old girl presents with vomiting and palsy. X-ray of the abdomen shows bilateral renal calcification.

Serum	Na	125	mmol/l
	K	2.3	mmol/l
	Cl	118	mmol/l
	SBC	12	mmol/l

Arterial	pH	7.20
Urine	pH	6.80

1. What is the acid-base disorder?
2. What is the clinical diagnosis?
3. How do you treat?
4. After treatment of acid-base disorder, what test can be performed to confirm diagnosis?

Question 5

An 18-year-old girl was admitted for diarrhoea.

Serum	Na	128	mmol/l	
	K	3.2	mmol/l	
	Cl	98	mmol/l	
	SBC	20	mmol/l	
	Creatinine	1.8	mg/dl	(159 µmol/l)
	Urea	126	mg/dl	(21 mmol/l)

Urine	Na	3	mmol/l	
	K	25	mmol/l	
	Osmolality	850	mOsmol/l	
	Creatinine	180	mg/dl	(159 µmol/l)

1. What is the status of patient's body water?
2. Why are plasma creatinine and urea elevated?
3. Would you give patient 3% saline?
4. Why is serum K^+ low?

Question 6

A 40-year-old man was admitted for dyspnoea, oedema and mitral valve disease.

Serum	A	B		Urine	A	B	
Na	123	135	mmol/l	Na	2	40	mmol/l
K	3.4	2.7	mmol/l	K	2.8	65	mmol/l
Cl	96	87	mmol/l	Creatinine	280	70	mg/dl
Creatinine	2.8	1.0	mg/dl	Osmolality	490	200	mOsmol/kg
Urea	120	40	mg/dl	24 hr vol	400	2000	ml
Osmolality	257	285	mOsmol/kg				

1. Does hyponatraermia at A indicate total body Na^+ deficit?
2. Why is the biochemistry different in A and B?
3. Why does he have hypokalaemia at A and why is it worse at B?
4. Why are serum creatinine and urea elevated?

Question 7

A 60-year-old man presents with cough and weight loss. Skin turgor is normal, neck veins are not distended and there is no oedema. Chest X-ray shows a right upper lobe density.

Serum	Na	124	mmol/l	
	K	3.7	mmol/l	
	Cl	88	mmol/l	
	SBC	24	mmol/l	
	Urea	8	mg/dl	(1.3 mmol/l)
	Creatinine	0.6	mg/dl	(53 µmol/l)
Urine	Na	39	mmol/l	
	Osmolality	340	mOsmol/kg	

1. What is his state of hydration?
2. Explain urinary Na^+ excretion and urine osmolality.

3. How do you treat this condition?
4. If serum urea was 160 mg/dl and creative 7.0 mg/dl would you change your diagnosis?

Question 8

A 48-year-old female had a hypophysectomy done to remove a pituitary adenoma. 72 hours later, she is confused and has lost 5 kg in weight (65 to 60 kg).

Serum	Na	165	mmol/l	
	K	4.3	mmol/l	
	Cl	132	mmol/l	
	SBC	24	mmol/l	
	Urea	56	mg/dl	(9.3 mmol/l)
	Creatinine	1.8	mg/dl	(159 μmol/l)
	Calcium	10.4	mg/dl	(2.6 mmol/l)

Urine	Na	4	mmol/l
	Osmolality	90	mOsmol/kg

1. Why is she hypernatraemic?
2. Explain increased creatinine, urine Na^+ and urine osmolality.
3. Calculate fluid deficit if there is no gain or loss of total body Na^+.
4. Treatment?

Question 9

A 23-year-old male had severe diarrhoea and fever. His weight is 50 kg.

Serum	Na	162	mmol/l
	K	4.0	mmol/l
	Cl	133	mmol/l
	SBC	18	mmol/l
	Hct	48	%
	Osmolality	327	mOsmol/l

1. How much saline do you give?
2. How much water to correct hypernatraemia?
3. What are the dangers of giving this as 5% dextrose and water very rapidly? Very slowly?
4. What fluid therapy would be best?

Question 10
A 57-year-old woman was admitted for syncopal attack and vomiting. She had a previous history of duodenal ulcer.

		Day 1	Day 5	
Arterial	pH	7.62	7.48	
	$PaCO_2$	75	36	mm Hg
	PaO_2	52	82	mm Hg
	SBC	75	26	mmol/l
Serum	Na	141	142	mmol/l
	K	1.8	4.3	mmol/l
	Cl	51	103	mmol/l

1. What is the acid-base disorder present?
2. Is compensation adequate?
3. What would you expect urine Cl⁻ to have been on Day 1?
4. Discuss treatment.

Question 11
A 50-year-old man was admitted in coma. He was cyanotic and febrile, barrel-chested and had finger clubbing. Chest X-ray showed a right lower lobe consolidation.

Arterial	pH	7.24	
	$PaCO_2$	91	mm Hg
	PaO_2	38	mm Hg
	SBC	38	mmol/l

Serum	Na	138	mmol/l
	K	5.0	mmol/l
	Cl	85	mmol/l

1. What is the acid-base disturbance present?
2. Is compensation adequate?
3. Comment on underlying disorder?
4. Treatment.

Question 12

An 18-year-old model was admitted for hyperventilation and confusion. She had been taking an unknown medication for 6 months to maintain her curvaceous figure.

		0 hours	6 hours	12 hours	
Arterial	pH	6.78	7.33	7.44	
	$PaCO_2$	14	19	28	mm Hg
	SBC	2	10	19	mmol/l
Serum	Na	144	146	151	mmol/l
	K	5.2	2.1	2.7	mmol/l
	Cl	137	118	119	mmol/l

1. What is the acid-base disorder at Time Zero?
2. Discuss differential diagnosis and treatment.
3. Explain lab values.
4. What happened to plasma K^+?

ANSWERS

Answer 1

1. He is dehydrated (salt depleted).

2. Serum osmolality $= (Na^+ \, K)\, 2 + \dfrac{glucose}{18} + \dfrac{urea}{6}$

$$= (157+2.3)\, 2 + \dfrac{238}{18} + \dfrac{360}{6}$$

$$= 392 \text{ mOsmol/kg}$$

NB: If glucose, urea is expressed as mmol/l, it is not necessary to divide by 18 and 6.

1. Diagnosis: Hyperosmolar non-ketotic diabetes.
2. Normal serum osmolality $= 285 \pm 5$ mOsmol/kg
3. Hypokalaemic metabolic alkalosis.
4. Treatment consists of normal saline infusion with potassium chloride replacement.

Answer 2

1. Metabolic Acidosis with salt depletion.
2. This is due to pre-renal failure resulting from dehydration.
3. Calculation of sodium deficit:
   (Normal serum Na^+ – patient's serum Na^+) $\times$ $\tfrac{2}{3}$ BW in kg
   Assuming normal serum Na^+ is 140 mEq/l,
   Sodium deficit $= (140 - 120) \times \tfrac{2}{3} \times 65 = 867$ mEq/l of sodium
4. Calculation of bicarbonate deficit:
   Assuming normal serum bicarbonate is 25 mEq/1,
   Deficit $= (25 - 10) \times \tfrac{1}{3} \times 65 = 325$ ml of 8.4% sodium bicarbonate.

Answer 3

1. Metabolic Acidosis.
2. Urine in bowels causes irritation inducing a villous diarrhoea.
3. Bicarbonate Deficit $= (25 - 15) \times \frac{1}{3} \times 60$
   $$= 10 \times 20 = 200 \text{ ml of } 8.4\% \text{ NaHCO}_3$$
4. Long-term complications are urinary infection and ureteric stenosis due to stricture at site of ureteric implantation into bowels. The stenosis can cause obstructive uropathy.

Answer 4

1. Hyperchloraemic metabolic acidosis.
2. Type I Renal Tubular Acidosis (RTA), also known as Distal or Classic Renal Tubular Acidosis (RTA). These patients have nephrocalcinosis and are still unable to acidify the urine in spite of severe metabolic acidosis, in contrast to patients with Type II or Proximal RTA.
3. Treatment consists of sodium bicarbonate together with potassium replacement.
4. Ammonium Chloride Loading Test can be performed.

Answer 5

1. Patient is dehydrated (salt and water depletion) as evidenced by history of watery diarrhoea and low serum sodium.
2. This is due to pre-renal failure resulting from diarrhoea.
3. No, this patient requires water as well as sodium, hence normal saline infusion is better than 3% saline.
4. Potassium is low because of secondary hyperaldosteronism. Dehydration stimulates increased aldosterone secretion. This causes increased sodium absorption and potassium excretion.

Answer 6

1. No, patient has dilutional hyponatraemia due to excess body water.
2. He was treated with diuretics.
3. He has diuretic induced hypokalaemia.
4. This is due to pre-renal failure.

Answer 7

1. The patient has excess water due to inappropriate secretion of antidiuretic hormone (SIADH).

   Excess water:
   Weight = 65 kg × 0.6 = 39 litres total body water
   Serum sodium = 124 mEq/l

   $$\frac{124}{140} \times 39 = 34.5 \text{ litres}$$

   39 − 34.5 = 4.5 litres excess water

2. In SIADH, the urine is concentrated, urine sodium is more than 20 mEq/l, hence urine osmolality is high (340 mOsmol/kg).
3. Treatment:
   i) Excretion of excess water:
      Use diuretics, replace electrolytes with IV hypertonic saline.
   ii) Oedematous hyponatraemic patient:
      Treat with sodium and water restriction. Agents that antagonize renal action of arginine vasopressin (AVP) like lithium and demeclochlorcycline can also be used. Recently, antagonist of hydro-osmotic effect of AVP has been introduced which causes water diuresis with no solute excretion.
4. Patient has renal failure with salt losing nephropathy.

Answer 8

1. She has no ADH and has lost much body water.
2. The patient has little sodium and low urinary osmolarity. This is due to a lack of ADH. ADH enables one to produce concentrated urine. A lack of it will cause the passage of very dilute urine.
3. Fluid deficit:
   Weight = 60 kg × 0.6 = 36 litres total body water.
   Water needed to lower serum sodium to 140 meq/l:

   $$\frac{165}{140} \times 36 = 42.4 \text{ litres}$$

   42.4 − 36 = 6.4 litres (water deficit).

4. Treatment consists of water or 5% dextrose.

Answer 9

1. No saline as patient has hypernatraemia.
2. Water required to correct hypernatraemia:
   Weight = 50 kg × 0.6 = 30 litres total body water
   Water needed to lower serum sodium to 140 mEq/l:

   $$\frac{162}{140} \times 30 = 34.7 \text{ litres}$$

   34.7 − 30 = 4.7 litres water.

3. If water or 5% dextrose is given too rapidly, patient may develop cerebral oedema. Given slowly, idiogenic osmoles have time to dissipate.
4. The best form of fluid therapy is ½ strength saline.

Answer 10

1. Respiratory acidosis and metabolic alkalosis.
2. Compensation:
   Rise in standard bicarbonate = 4 × (rise in $PaCO_2$) ± 4 mmol/l = 4 × ($\frac{35}{10}$) ± 4 = 14 mmol/l.
   But patient's SBC is 75 mmol/l, compensation is more than adequate.
3. Urine chloride is expected to be high because of paradoxical aciduria.
4. Treatment consists of oxygen and I.V. normal saline.

Answer 11

1. Chronic respiratory acidosis with acute hypercapnia.
2. Compensation:
   Compensation of SBC should rise above 24 mmol/l by 4 mmol/l per 10 mm Hg increment in $paCO_2$ above 40 mm Hg within a range of ± 4 mmol/l.

   $$\text{ie. Rise in SBC} = 4 \times \frac{\text{rise in } PaCO_2}{10}$$

   $$= (4 \times \tfrac{50}{10}) \pm 4 = 16 \text{ mmol/l}$$

   Patient's SBC is 18 mmol/l. Compensation is therefore adequate.

   In Respiratory Acidosis:
   > There is increased $PaCO_2$ (> 40 mm Hg)
   > Arterial pH is decreased (Acidaemia)
   > SBC is high (compensation)
   > Low Serum Chloride
   > Serum K is normal or low.

3. This patient has a chronic obstructive airway disease with pneumonia and respiratory failure.
4. Adequate oxygen and treatment of underlying cause.

Answer 12

1. Severe Metabolic Acidosis with Compensatory Respiratory Alkalosis.
2. The patient may have taken aspirin, inducing metabolic acidosis and treated with forced alkaline diuresis using bicarbonate, normal saline infusion and frusemide.
3. Explanation of lab values:
   This is the result of the above treatment as well as correction by respiratory compensation.

   Compensation:
   $PaCO_2 = 14$, SBC = 2
   $PaCO_2 = (1.5 \times SBC) + 8 \pm 2$
   $\qquad = 11 \pm 2$ mm Hg

   Value for $PaCO_2$ below 9 or above 13 defines mixed disturbance.
4. Plasma K is low because of loss in the urine due to forced diuresis. As acidosis is corrected, patient tends towards alkalosis, and plasma K also falls.

Additional Notes

Respiratory Alkalosis accounts for 46% of all acid-base disorders.

There is decreased $PaCO_2$ (< 40 mm Hg)
Arterial pH is high (alkalaemia)
SBC is low (compensation)
High serum chloride

In Respiratory Alkalosis:

$PaCO_2$ is seldom below 14 mmol/l (range 14 to 24) and SBC seldom less than 18 mmol/l.
Normal: $PaCO_2 = 40$ mm Hg
$\qquad$ SBC $= 25$ mmol/l

Treatment:

 i. Oxygen if hypoxaemic.
 ii. Treat volume depletion, hypotension, sepsis.
iii. If pH > 7.55, anaesthetise, ventilate and paralyse patient. This is the best means of raising $PaCO_2$ and decreasing pH in severe alkalaemia.

+ Table 16.1   Simple acid-base disorders*

Type of Disorder	pH	$PaCO_2$	$[HCO_3^-]$
Metabolic acidosis	↓	↓	↓
Metabolic alkalosis	↑	↑	↑
Acute respiratory acidosis	↓	↑	↑
Chronic respiratory acidosis	↓	↑	↑
Acute respiratory alkalosis	↑	↓	↓
Chronic respiratory alkalosis	↑	↓	↓

Note that the metabolic ($[HCO_3^-]$ and respiratory ($PaCO_2$) components of the "acid-base equation" always change in the same direction in simple acid-base disorders.
+ Courtesy of R. Schrier.

+ Table 16.2 Rules of thumb for bedside interpretation of Acid-Base Disorders

Metabolic acidosis	$PaCO_2$ should fall by 1.0 to 1.5 × the fall in plasma HCO_3^- concentration.
Metabolic alkalosis	$PaCO_2$ should rise by 0.25 to 1.0 × the rise in plasma HCO_3^- concentration.
Acute respiratory acidosis	Plasma HCO_3^- concentration should rise by about 1 mmol/l for each 10 mm Hg increment in $PaCO_2$ (±3 mmol/l).
Chronic respiratory acidosis	Plasma HCO_3^- concentration should rise by about 4 mmol/l for each 10 mm Hg increment in $PaCO_2$ (±4 mmol/l)
Acute respiratory alkalosis	Plasma HCO_3^- concentration should fall by about 1–3 mmol/l for each 10 mm Hg decrement in the $PaCO_2$ usually not to less than 18 mmol/l.
Chronic respiratory alkalosis	Plasma HCO_3^- concentration should fall by about 2–5 mmol/l per 10 mm Hg decrement in $PaCO_2$ but usually not to less than 14 mmol/l.

+ *Courtesy of R. Schrier.*

CHAPTER 17

Renal Tubular Acidosis

Renal tubular acidosis (RTA) is a clinical syndrome of disordered renal acidification characterised by minimal or no azotaemia, hyperchloracmic acidosis, inappropriately high urinary pH, bicarbonaturia and reduced urinary excretion of titratable acid (TA) and ammonium (NH_4^+). The syndrome reflects a disorder of renal acidification that can cause acidosis with little or no apparent reduction in renal mass as measured by the glomerular filtration rate (GFR).

Renal tubular acidosis was first described by Lightwood and Butler in children and by Baines et al in the adult. Two main types of RTA have been described (Types I and II), though at least four types have now been recognised (Types III and IV).

TYPE I RTA

Type I RTA, also known as Distal or Classic RTA is due to an inability of the distal tubule to establish an adequate pH gradient between the blood and the distal tubular fluid. There is a defect in the luminal membrane causing a limitation of tubular cell lumen H^+ gradient. Type I RTA per se is not associated with impaired tubular reabsorption of amino acids or glucose. Even during severe degrees of acidosis the urine pH does not drop below 5.4, in contrast to Type II RTA. Furthermore tubular reabsorption of bicarbonate in the proximal tubule is not greatly reduced. The defect is due to an inability to generate or maintain normally steep lumen-peritubular H^+ gradients. A significant disposal of H^+ ions as titratable acid and ammonium is possible provided the distal tubule can achieve a large H^+ ion gradient. When the distal tubule is incapable of transporting H^+ ion efficiently the urine pH remains more alkaline than would be expected and the plasma bicarbonate falls. Characteristically, these patients have hyperchloraemic acidosis, often accompanied by hypokalaemia, normal glomerular filtration rates and a tendency to develop nephrocalcinosis and renal calculi.

Type I RTA, like Type II RTA, can be primary (idiopathic) or secondary, ie. due to exogenous causes or associated with other renal or generalised disorder. In a series of 10 cases, Type I RTA seems to be the one we encounter. Six of the 10 cases had secondary RTA: 2 due to medullary sponge kidney, 2 associated with gout, 1 with idiopathic hypercalciuria and hyperuricosuria and the remaining associated with systemic lupus erythematosus. Other causes of secondary Type I RTA are described in association with hypercalcaemia, light chain proteinuria, amphotericin toxicity, toluene toxicity (glue or paint sniffing), lithium toxicity and transplant rejection. Primary RTA can be genetically transmitted as an autosomal dominant trait or it can occur sporadically.

Medullary sponge kidney is a disease characterised by collecting ductular ectasia. It affects primarily the papillary portion of the medulla. Disorder of tubular function has been described with medullary sponge kidney and it consists of an inability of the kidney to concentrate and acidify the urine maximally, ie. a distal or Type I RTA.

The occurrence of RTA in patients with medullary sponge kidney and Ehlers-Danlos syndrome has led workers to suggest that the acidification defect reflects a structural rather than a metabolic defect. The acidification defect might of course result from a metabolic abnormality of the epithelial membrane. In medullary sponge disease the impairment in renal acidification may be the result of structural alterations of the renal tubule initiated by deposition of calcium salts in the renal parenchyma. This possibility is suggested by the association of Type I RTA and nephrocalcinosis in a variety of clinical conditions in which Type I RTA is not a characteristic complication in the absence of nephrocalcinosis: primary hyperparathyroidism, vitamin D intoxication, hyperthyroidism, idiopathic hypercalciuria and medullary sponge kidney.

In 1959 Wrong and Davis described a form of RTA without overt metabolic acidosis. They suggested that such patients had an incomplete RTA which could be preacidotic. In our series we had 2 patients who initially presented with nephrocalcinosis, normal plasma bicarbonate, a marked acidification defect and a normal production of ammonia. It is important to detect this type of Incomplete Type I RTA because like the complete form, renal calcification and osteomalacia may disappear with long-term alkali therapy.

TYPE II RTA

The other main type of RTA is Type II RTA which is also referred to as Proximal RTA. These patients have a defect in the reabsorption of bicarbonate by the proximal tubule that causes the distal tubule to be flooded with bicarbonate. If the plasma bicarbonate is low or lowered by the prolonged use of ammonium chloride, the reduced filtered load of bicarbonate can be reabsorbed, allowing the final urine to fall to normal acid levels. This group of patients who often have other evidence of proximal tubular involvement such as aminoaciduria, phosphaturia and glycosuria usually require larger amounts of alkali to correct their acidosis than do those who have the distal tubular defect (Type I RTA). Type II RTA is associated with certain errors of metabolism (cystinosis, Wilson's disease) or it can be a consequence of heavy metal toxicity, outdated tetracycline, multiple myeloma, dysproteinaemia, nephrotic syndrome or transplant rejection. A mild form may be seen in primary or secondary hyperparathyroidism.

Type II RTA also exists in an incomplete form. These are patients with Fanconi's Syndrome who are not acidotic, ie. net renal secretion of H^+ at normal plasma bicarbonate was not subnormal. They resemble Incomplete Type I RTA, except urinary pH decreases to appropriate low values during Ammonium Chloride Loading.

TYPE III RTA

Type III RTA has been referred to as a Dislocation or Bicarbonate Wasting "Classic" RTA which presents as a bicarbonate wasting RTA that is not Fanconi's syndrome (triad of proximal tubular dysfunction of renal glycosuria, aminoaciduria and increased phosphate clearance).

TYPE IV RTA

In this type of RTA, patients with Chronic Renal Insufficiency become acidotic before the GFR becomes greatly reduced (ie. before 30 ml/ min). The pathology in this group of patients does not affect the glomeruli principally, rather it is associated with tubulo-interstitial diseases like reflux nephropathy, polycystic kidney and analgesic nephropathy. These patients have hyporeninaemia and hypoaldosteronism, while their acidosis is usually associated with hyperchloraemia, hyperkalaemia and acidic urine. Their physiology is like those of Type II (Proximal) RTA with 2–17% bicarbonaturia. However they do not have features of Fanconi's syndrome. It is postulated that they have a combined defect in secretion of H^+ and K^+ in the distal tubule and the cause could be a deficiency or a resistance to the action of aldosterone.

There were 2 patients in our series who initially presented with Incomplete Type I RTA as evidenced by impaired urinary acidification in the absence of systemic acidosis. Their plasma bicarbonate levels were 24 and 25 mEq/l. In these patients, systemic acidosis is not present and net acid excretion does not appear to be frankly subnormal, although urinary pH is clearly inappropriately high when measured during ammonium chloride induced acidosis.

INVESTIGATIONS

1. Blood urea, serum creatinine, electrolytes, serum bicarbonate
2. Blood gases
3. Urine pH
4. Ammonium Chloride Loading Test
5. Maximal Osmolar Concentration
6. 24-hour urinary calcium, uric acid
7. 24-hour urinary amino acids, phosphate; glycosuria
8. Serum calcium, phosphate and serum alkaline phosphatase, serum uric acid
9. Urinary protein, Creatinine Clearance Test
10. Radiological: X-ray abdomen, intravenous pyelogram, tomogram, skeletal survey
11. Collagen work-up: ESR, ANF, anti-DNA, serum immunoglobulins, serum complement

Ammonium Chloride Loading Test

Patients were allowed to have a light breakfast before onset of test and at 8 am, oral NH_4 Cl was given in a dose of 0.1 gm/kg BW with a cup of orange juice or plain water. Urine was voided at 8 am and discarded, following which all urine passed from 8 am till 10 am was collected and labelled as First Specimen. At 10 am a blood gas was done. Urine from 1 pm to 3 pm was again collected and this was labelled as Second Specimen. A specimen of arterial blood was again collected for blood gas analysis.

Patients who were unable to acidify the urine to a pH of 5.3 at the Second Specimen were considered to have an impairment of urinary acidification. Urinary specimens were estimated for the following:

	lst specimen	2nd specimen
• pH of urine	4.75–5.5	4.5–5.2
• Titratable Acid	14.4–39 mEq/min	14.6–34.4 mEq/min
• Ammonium (NH_4^+)	39–154 mEq/min	39–58 mEq/min

Maximal Osmolar Concentration

Patients were put on a fast from midnight and on arrival at the ward the next day a subcutaneous injection of pitressin tannate in oil (5 units) was administered at 8 am. Urine was then collected at hourly intervals from 9 am onwards, both the volume as well as the osmolarity being measured at the same time. The test was terminated after 6 to 8 samples of urine had been collected or if the urine osmolarity had already exceeded 800 mOsmol/l, whichever occurred first. The highest concentration reached during this period would be the Maximal Osmolar Concentration (MOC) and a concentration defect was said to be present if the MOC was less than 800 mOsmol/l at the end of the test period.

The normal ranges for some of the indices measured above are as follows:

1. 24-hour urinary amino acid
   normal adult male   = 2.9–12.5 mmol/day   40–175 mg/day
   normal adult female   = 2.1–9.5 mmol/day   29–133 mg/day
2. 24–hour urinary inorganic phosphate
   adult male   = 6.5–32.3 mmol/day   0.2–1.0 gm/day
   adult female   = 8.1–22.6 mmol/day   0.25–0.7 gm/day
3. 24-hour urinary calcium
   adult male   = 0.41–3.38 mmol/day   33–270 mg/day
   adult female   = 0.33–3.13 mmol/day   26–250 mg/day
4. 24-hour urinary uric acid = up to 4.2 mmol/day   700 mg/day

TYPE I OR DISTAL RTA
(Classic or Gradient RTA)

This is due to a defect in the distal tubule whereby it is unable to generate a sufficient hydrogen ion gradient to cause its secretion into the distal tubular lumen. The excretion of titratable acid (TA) and ammonium (NH_4^+) therefore will be low and the urine pH remains alkaline (above 5.3). The patient will not be able to acidify the urine despite severe metabolic acidosis (serum bicarbonate < 15 mEq/1) unlike Type II RTA.

Clinical Features of Type I RTA

1. The commonest mode of presentation is muscular weakness or paralysis due to hypokalaemia. Some patients present with haematuria or renal colic due to renal calculi. Urinary tract infection may complicate renal stones and occasionally,

obstructive uropathy with renal failure may result. Properly treated, these patients should not develop renal failure.

2. A low serum K^+ associated with hyperchloraemia and metabolic acidosis should alert one to the possibility of the patient having RTA. The differential diagnosis is a patient with an ileal conduit or ureterosigmoidostomy. If the patient has renal failure, then RTA cannot be diagnosed and the acidosis is likely to be due to uraemic acidosis in which case the serum K^+ is usually high.

   Urine pH and blood gases should be performed when RTA is suspected. In the presence of severe acidosis and urine pH more than 5.3 with hypokalaemia and hyperchloraemia, a diagnosis of Type I RTA is fairly certain. The presence of nephrocalcinosis on plain X-ray of the abdomen confirms the diagnosis of Type I RTA as patients with Type II RTA do not usually have nephrocalcinosis. Patients with Type II RTA are able to acidify the urine (pH less than 5.3) when acidosis is severe (serum bicarbonate less than 15 mEq/l).

3. A skeletal survey should be performed in patients with RTA as children may have rickets and adults osteomalacia. Rickets is due to low serum calcium resulting from failure of the renal tubules to produce adequate amounts of 1,25-dihydroxycholecalciferol. Some patients have osteomalacia because of low serum phosphate. This occurs in those with Type II RTA because of associated phosphaturia.

TYPE II OR PROXIMAL RTA
(Bicarbonate Wasting or Rate RTA)

The defect is in the proximal tubule whereby there is an inability to reabsorb filtered bicarbonate. Normally, the proximal tubule reabsorbs up to 85% of filtered bicarbonate, the distal tubule about 10 to 15% and the collecting duct about 5%. In Type II RTA only about 65% of bicarbonate is reabsorbed. The excess bicarbonate (about 35%) is now presented at the distal tubule. But this is much more than what the distal tubule can absorb. Excess bicarbonate therefore remains in the urine and keeps it alkaline (urine pH > 5.3).

However, when the patient is severely acidotic, the little bicarbonate presented at the proximal tubule is almost completely reabsorbed. Only a little filters into the distal tubule. Since the distal tubular mechanism is intact in Proximal RTA and there is now no excess bicarbonate to compete for excretion of titratable acid and ammonium, the distal tubular acidification proceeds normally and urine is acidified with urine *pH* of less than 5.3.

The patient with Proximal RTA also has associated features of glycosuria, aminoaciduria, hypophosphataemia and hypouricaemia in addition to the usual features of RTA like hypokalaemia, hyperchloraemic acidosis and alkaline urine as in Type I RTA.

Each time bicarbonate is reabsorbed, whether by the proximal or distal tubule, it is accompanied by the reabsorption of sodium (Na^+). The reabsorption of Na^+ is accompanied by excretion of either H^+ or K^+. Normally H^+ is excreted in the form of titratable acid and ammonium. If bicarbonate is not reabsorbed, Na^+ is not absorbed and H^+ is not excreted. The result is metabolic acidosis. In addition, patients with Type II RTA also have a reduction in the rate of H^+ secretion into the tubular lumen. K^+ is therefore excreted in exchange for reabsorbed Na^+ and hence patients become hypokalaemic.

In Type I or distal RTA, since H^+ cannot be secreted, K^+ is exchanged with Na^+ absorption and the patient develops hypokalaemic acidosis.

In many patients with Proximal RTA due to Fanconi's syndrome, renal acidification defect involves both the proximal and the distal tubule.

Clinical Features of Type II or Proximal RTA

1. The clinical manifestations of hypokalaemic paralysis and metabolic acidosis are the same as those of Type I RTA. Patients with Type II RTA have a triad of proximal tubular dysfunction of renal glycosuria, aminoaciduria and increased phosphate clearance (low serum phosphate). Serum uric acid is often low (less than 2 mg/dl) because of associated hypouricaemia. If they have associated distal tubular defects (Type I RTA) as many patients with Fanconi's syndrome do, they will also have nephrocalcinosis with renal stones, colic and haematuria with occasional urinary infection due to stones.

2. These patients are able to acidify the urine when acidosis is severe (serum bicarbonate < 15 mEq/l) because the distal tubule is intact. The urine pH will then be < 5.3 instead of about 7 or 8.

3. Skeletal survey may show rickets or osteomalacia.

TREATMENT OF RTA

1. Treatment will vary with the type of RTA and the underlying cause. Patients with Type I RTA require less bicarbonate than those with Type II RTA who may require as much as 10 to 20 gm of bicarbonate, hence the term "bicarbonate wasting RTA". Patients with Type II RTA usually require more than 6 mEq/kg/day of bicarbonate in contrast to those with Type I where they require much less (about 1.5 mEq/kg/day).

2. Hypokalaemia will require potassium chloride replacement. KCl should be given slowly in a continuous intravenous drip. Oral supplements can also be given. Patients with Type II RTA usually require much more KCl for correction of hypokalaemia and they usually require maintenance KCl supplements even when acidosis has been corrected.

3. Patients should be encouraged to drink a lot of fluids as this has been shown to be helpful in reducing nephrocalcinosis. Their fluid regimen should be the same as for anyone with stones, ie. to drink especially before retiring to bed so that he would wake up in the night to pass urine and thereafter to drink again to pass once more in the early morning. Patients should drink enough to pass at least 3 litres of urine a day.

4. Vitamin D therapy (1,25 dihydroxycholecalciferol) and calcium supplements are necessary if they have rickets or osteomalacia.

5. A 24-hour urinary estimate of calcium and uric acid should be performed to exclude idiopathic hypercalciuria and hyperuricosuria as such patients may require treatment with thiazides and allopurinol if they do not respond to dietary counselling.

6. Finally, energetic treatment should be promptly instituted for those who develop obstructive uropathy (due to calculus disease) and urinary infections.

7. With proper management, renal failure should never occur in patients with RTA.

PRACTICE POINTS

1. If nephrocalcinosis is present the patient is likely to have Type I RTA.

2. If the patient has severe acidosis (serum bicarbonate < 15 mEq/l) and cannot acidify the urine (urine pH > 5.3)

he has Type I RTA. There is no necessity in performing the ammonium chloride test.

3. A patient with Type I RTA cannot acidify the urine, ie. bring the urine pH down to < 5.3, no matter how acidotic he is, unlike one with Type II RTA where the distal tubule is intact and can secrete H^+ into the urine.

4. The ammonium chloride loading test should not be performed when the patient is acidotic.

5. In performing the ammonium chloride loading test, it is necessary to do a blood gas and confirm that the patient has systemic acidosis. If he is not acidotic it may mean that he has vomited the ammonium chloride which would render the test useless unless he takes another dose.

CHAPTER 18

Renal Tubular Disorders

The following conditions can cause renal tubular disorders:

1. Renal Tubular Acidosis (RTA): Type I or Distal RTA
2. Fanconi's syndrome: Type II or Proximal RTA
3. Cystinuria
4. Cystinosis
5. Medullary sponge kidney
6. Medullary cystic kidney
7. Diabetes insipidus
8. Pseudohypoparathyroidism
9. Uraemic acidosis
10. Interstitial nephritis

Renal Tubular Acidosis and Fanconi's Syndrome have been covered in the chapter on Renal Tubular Acidosis.

CYSTINURIA

1. This is a proximal tubular lesion. It is usually inherited in an autosomal recessive manner but can occasionally be autosomal dominant.
2. Patients are unable to reabsorb cystine, ornithine, lysine and arginine. These 4 amino acids can be remembered by C.O.L.A.
3. It is associated with small bowel disturbance where the same amino acids are also not absorbed. There may be a common transport disorder.

4. Renal calculi is the usual manifestation. These stones are radio opaque as they contain sulphur.
5. Treatment consists of alkalinisation of the urine, diuretics and in severe cases, penicillamine. Penicillamine itself causes side effects like gastrointestinal upset, liver dysfunction and nephrotic syndrome.

CYSTINOSIS

1. This condition is due to an accumulation of cystine in the reticuloendothelial system, leukocytes, fibroblasts, kidneys and eyes
2. One should look for crystals in the lymph node, leukocyte, bone marrow, cornea (using slit lamp), and kidneys.
3. It is a cause of Fanconi's syndrome causing Type II or proximal RTA. The childhood form is associated with growth failure and renal failure because of its severity.
4. Retinopathy due to cystine deposits in the retina may cause blindness.
5. The adult type is more benign as the kidneys can be spared. However, a variant exists which occurs as a late onset juvenile type and such patients may have slow progressive renal failure.
6. Patients with cystinosis with Fanconi's syndrome have aminoaciduria, glycosuria and rickets. Cystine stones are rare.

MEDULLARY SPONGE KIDNEY

1. This is a congenital condition related to an abnormality of the collecting duct of the kidney where there is dilatation of the renal tubules (tubuloectasia), sometimes "cystic", which communicates with the calyces.

2. Patients may present with haematuria, urinary tract infection related to stones or nephrocalcinosis. They may also present as Type I RTA with nephrocalcinosis.
3. The diagnosis may be suspected by the pattern of nephrocalcinosis and stones on a plain film of the abdomen. An IVP confirms the diagnosis.
4. An ammonium chloride loading test and maximal osmolar concentration are usually performed to exclude RTA and assess tubular function. It is also useful to measure the 24-hour urinary excretion of calcium and uric acid as there is an association with idiopathic hypercalciuria and hyperuricosuria.
5. Treatment consists of drinking enough fluids to pass at least 3 litres of urine a day. Urinary infections and stones should be treated.

MEDULLARY CYSTIC KIDNEYS

1. This disease is inherited in an autosomal recessive fashion.
2. Patients have a congenital cystic dilatation of the tubules.
3. They may present with cramps and hypotension due to salt loss resulting from impaired tubular function.
4. Anaemia, polyuria and acidosis are common presentations related to chronic renal failure which most would have by the time they become juveniles. They are also stunted because of renal bone disease.
5. A non-specific aminoaciduria may also be associated as a manifestation of Type II RTA which can be diagnosed only when the patient still has normal renal function.
6. This is a condition with a poor prognosis unlike medullary sponge kidneys which have a good prognosis and is compatible with normal life expectancy.

DIABETES INSIPIDUS (DI)

1. May be neurogenic (Pituitary DI) or nephrogenic (Nephrogenic DI) in origin.

   In Pit DI the renal tubules are normal but the pituitary fails to produce antidiuretic hormone (ADH) and the urine therefore is not concentrated and the patient has frequency of micturition associated with polyuria.

   In Nephrogenic DI there is ADH but the tubules are not capable of responding to ADH and therefore the urine is always hypotonic to plasma. Patients also have increased frequency of micturition and polyuria.

2. In Pit DI the onset is often acute with increased frequency of micturition, especially at night, every half to one hour; whereas in Nephrogenic DI the onset is more gradual.

   Cerebrovascular disease is a common cause of Pit DI, especially in elderly patients. In about 30% of Pit DI the cause is unknown.

   Nephrogenic DI may be congenital or drug induced, eg. lithium given for depression. Other causes include hypokalaemia, hypercalcaemia as well as hydronephrosis and pyelonephritis where damage to the distal tubules results in their failure to respond to ADH.

3. A Pitressin Test (Maximal Osmolar Concentration) can help to differentiate Pit DI from Nephrogenic DI. In Pit DI there will be a response to pitressin and one of the urine specimens will show an osmolarity > 800 mosmol/l, but in Nephrogenic DI there will be no response to pitressin. In a patient with normal plasma osmolarity of 285 mosmol/l and urine osmolarity of 140 to 180 mosmol/l not responding to pitressin, the diagnosis is Nephrogenic DI.

One should be very very cautious in performing the Pitressin test in the elderly as there is the risk of inducing a stroke or a myocardial infarction. Do a baseline ECG and assess for cerebrovascular insufficiency before proceeding if one must perform the test in an elderly patient.

4. Treatment consists of removal of the underlying cause. In Nephrogenic DI thiazides are useful. They cause increased excretion of Na+ at the distal tubule. This stimulates proximal tubular reabsorption of Na+ and water, and less fluid is delivered to the distal tubule to be excreted. The electrolytes and renal function must be monitored, especially in the elderly. In Pit DI chlorpropamide may be useful as it has a "pitressin-like effect" on cyclic AMP on the distal tubule. The blood sugar must be monitored because of the risk of hypoglycaemia. Desmopressin or intranasal pitressin can also be used, but with caution in the elderly.

PSEUDOHYPOPARATHYROIDISM

1. These patients have the characteristic shortened 4th metacarpal.
2. The biochemical features consist of low serum calcium due to decreased absorption from the bowels. They have a high serum phosphate.
3. Hypocalciuria and hypophosphaturia are additional features of the condition.

URAEMIC ACIDOSIS

1. Irrespective of the cause, Chronic Progressive Renal Disease results in some degree of systemic acidosis when the GFR is less than 25 ml/min. This is due to:

   i. impaired reabsorption of bicarbonate

   ii. impaired production of ammonia so that excretion of H^+ in the urine in the form of ammonium is decreased.

2. In some patients, there is a large amount of bicarbonate loss (ranging from 15% to as much as 50%) resembling bicarbonate wastage in Type II or Proximal RTA.

3. Part of the cause of the acidosis is related to the renal disease which reduces the activity of renal carbonic anhydrase. This enzyme is responsible for the generation of bicarbonate:

$$CO_2 + H_2O \xrightarrow{\text{Carbonic Anhydrase}} H_2CO^3$$

4. Seldin and Rector suggested that the impairment of bicarbonate reabsorption was a consequence of reduction in the number of functioning nephrons leading to reduced bicarbonate level.

5. Muldowny designated uraemic acidosis as parathyroid acidosis as he found the plasma concentration of parathormone was inversely correlated with plasma concentration of bicarbonate and hence the degree of systemic acidosis; ie. the higher the PTH levels the lower the serum bicarbonate level.

INTERSTITIAL NEPHRITIS

This is a term given to conditions where the main reaction of the kidney occurs in the interstitium. There is cellular reaction (usually lymphocytic) in the interstitium and tubular damage (atrophy and necrosis).

There are two types of Interstitial Nephritis:

I. Acute Interstitial Nephritis

1. Sudden onset usually due to:
   i. Drugs like non-steroidal anti-inflammatory drugs (NSAID), methicillin, ampicillin, sulphonamides, septrin, dilantin, dindevan, gentamicin, cephaloridine, allopurinol.
   ii. Septicaemia from any cause: leptospirosis, streptococcal and staphylococcal infection, cytomegalo-virus (CMV) infection.
   iii. Other causes include lupus nephritis, transplant rejection, beestings, toxins and poisons.
2. Antibiotics like methicillin, or even ampicillin can cause an acute allergic interstitial nephritis where the patient presents with fever, rash, haematuria (even gross haematuria), pyuria, proteinuria and acute renal failure with eosinophils in the urine.
   In a patient with acute allergic interstitial nephritis a renal biopsy would show interstitial oedema with infiltration of lymphocytes, plasma cells, polymorphs, eosinophils and varying degree of tubular atrophy and necrosis. The glomeruli are normal.
3. Treatment of acute interstitial nephritis consists of the removal of the offending drug and treating the infection. In the case of patients with acute renal failure they will require dialysis to tide them over the acute episode. For patients with acute allergic interstitial nephritis, prednisolone may be required.

II. Chronic Interstitial Nephritis

1. For this category of interstitial nephritis there is more interstitial fibrosis associated with chronic lymphocytic infiltrates and tubular atrophy.

2. The causes are:
   i. analgesic nephropathy, reflux nephropathy, polycystic kidneys.
   ii. chronic transplant rejection, lupus nephritis and chronic conditions like sarcoidosis
   iii. Sjogren's syndrome, irradiation, gout
   iv. lead and cadmium nephrotoxicity
   v. obstructive uropathy, heat stroke and medullary cystic kidneys
3. Treatment consists of removal or treatment of the underlying cause. A patient with analgesic nephropathy who stops taking analgesics will arrest the progression of the interstitial lesions.

CHAPTER 19

Systemic Disease and the Kidney

Considering that the kidneys receive about one quarter of the cardiac output and the glomeruli act as filters for blood constituents, it is not surprising that the kidneys are involved in various kinds of systemic diseases.

This chapter discusses the renal aspects of different types of systemic diseases.

RENAL VASCULITIS[1]

Vasculitis refers to necrotising inflammation of the blood vessels and is seen in a large spectrum of diseases. It could be due to any one of the following causes: some are systemic vasculitis and others predominantly renal vasculitis with a high incidence of end stage renal failure.

1. SLE
2. Polyarteritis nodosa (PAN)
3. Wegener's granulomatosis
4. Dermatomyositis
5. Henoch-Schonlein purpura
6. Cryoglobulinaemia
7. Rheumatoid arthritis
8. Hypersensitivity vasculitis
9. Behcet's disease

10. Infections: Hepatitis B antigen (positive in 6–40% of PAN), Beta-haemolytic strep, otitis media, post-infectious GN
11. Drugs: Sulphonamides, septrin, penicillin, iodine
12. Cancer: Leukaemia, lymphoma

Clinical Features

1. The peak age is between 40 to 50 years.
2. Patients often have a prodrome consisting of a flu-like illness. Some may have sores or history of drug ingestion.
3. Renal presentation could be haematuria, proteinuria, nephrotic syndrome, oliguria with acute renal failure or renal impairment.
4. Skin lesions such as purpura and cutaneous vasculitis.
5. Ocular lesions such as conjunctivitis, iritis.
6. Hypertension occurs in 25% of patients.
7. Liver, pancreas and gastrointestinal involvement with gastrointestinal bleeding and pain. These occur in 50% of patients.
8. CNS involvement occurs in 25% of patients: peripheral neuropathy is not uncommon.
9. Cardiovascular complications such as myocardial ischaemia and congestive heart failure.
10. Respiratory involvement may be in the form of bronchial asthma.

Investigation

1. ESR, FBC, Eosinophilia
2. LE cell, ANF, Anti-DNA
3. Serum complements, circulating immune complexes (CIC)
4. Cryoglobulinaemia

5. ASOT, Hepatitis B screening
6. Splanchnic or renal arteriogram to detect aneurysms

Renal Lesions

1. Glomerular
   i. Segmental necrotising glomerulitis, ischaemic shrinkage of glomeruli, glomerular fibrinoid necrosis, "segmental crescents".
   ii. Associated with mesangial proliferative GN, membranous GN, mesangiocapillary GN, endocapillary GN.
2. Tubular
   i. Acute tubular necrosis, interstitial lesions, infiltrate of plasma cells, lymphocytes, polymorphs.
   ii. Eosinophils present if vasculitis due to allergic angiitis and granulomatosis.
3. Renal blood vessels
   i. Fibrinoid necrosis with infiltration of polymorphs, eosinophils, lymphocytes.
   ii. Irregular intimal thickening, aneurysms, involving arcuate or interlobular arterial lesions.
4. IMF: Look for fibrin ++. Immunoglobulin staining depends on underlying cause.
5. EM features: Features depend on underlying cause.

Treatment

1. Prednisolone (1 mg/kg BW per day).
2. Cyclosphosphamide (2 mg/kg BW per day).
3. Pulse therapy with methylprednisolone (0.5 gm I.V. daily for 3 days).
4. Plasmapheresis has been shown to be useful in patients with rapidly progressive GN.

5. Dialysis is necessary in patients with oliguria, especially when they have more than 70% crescents on biopsy.
6. After renal transplantation, these patients have a low recurrence rate.

SYSTEMIC LUPUS ERYTHEMATOSUS

This has been dealt with separately in the chapter on Lupus Nephritis.

POLYARTERITIS NODOSA

This is a disease associated with fever, symptoms referrable to the muscles, gastrointestinal tract, lungs, heart and the kidneys. It is characterised by nodular swellings of medium-sized arteries.

Like SLE it has protean manifestations. Males are more commonly affected than females. All ages are affected. There is fever, leukocytosis, eosinophilia especially among patients with respiratory involvement, and is associated with weakness and weight loss. Patients may have arthritis, abdominal pain, polyneuritis, cardiac failure, asthma and pneumonia.

Renal involvement occurs in 70% of patients. They may present with acute nephritis with haematuria and proteinuria, sometimes with rapidly progressive glomerulonephritis. Others have only haematuria or proteinuria with rising serum creatinine. Some may develop malignant hypertension due to renal infarction and may have hypertensive cardiac failure. Death could result from cerebral haemorrhage or renal failure.

Renal arteriogram may show aneurysms affecting the larger arteries of the kidneys. Hepatitis B antigen has been associated with this condition.

The kidneys may be normal or reduced in size. There may be evidence of infarction. Petichial haemorrhages are associated with malignant hypertension. Small localised swellings may be seen on the main divisions of the renal artery in 70% of patients.

The renal biopsy changes include fibrinoid necrosis within the glomeruli. Epithelial crescents may be present. Part of the circumference of the blood vessels or the whole circumference may be replaced by fibrinoid necrosis. Plasma cells and sometimes eosinophils are found in the interstitium.

Treatment consists of prednisolone and cyclophosphamide. Plasmapheresis or methylprednisolone pulsing is usually prescribed for patients with rapidly progressive glomerulonephritis.

WEGENER'S GRANULOMATOSIS

Clinically, this condition is characterised by the presence of a granulomatous process in the upper respiratory tract and the lungs. The process is associated with necrosed blood vessels and a florid form of renal lesion in which the glomeruli show necrosis. About two-thirds of patients have purulent rhinorrhoea with nasal obstruction and crusting, antral pain, epistaxis while one-third has cough, haemoptysis and pleurisy.

The renal lesions are the same as for the microscopic form of polyarteritis nodosa, except that "granulomas" may form in relation to blood vessels, glomeruli and tubulo-interstitium. Rapidly progressive glomerulonephritis is associated with acute renal failure and the presence of crescents in the renal biopsy (pauci-immune crescenteric GN).

80% to 90% of patients are positive for cytoplasmic — anti neutrophilic cytoplasmic antibody (c-ANCA), which is highly specific and sensitive in the diagnosis. If untreated there is 80–90% mortality. Those treated with Cyclophosphamide have 80–90% remission. There is a high incidence of Cancer of the Bladder 10 years later in those treated with Cyclophosphamide. Prednisolone is used as adjunctive therapy especially for severe renal pulmonary, skin or cerebral vasculitis.

SCLERODERMA

This is also known as progressive systemic sclerosis. Males are more commonly affected than females with a predominance in the age group of 30 to 50 years.

Patients have calcinosis of the finger pulps on X-rays, Raynaud's phenomenon, sclerodactyly and telangiectasia (CRST syndrome).

Renal involvement occurs in about 45% of patients manifesting as proteinuria, hypertension, renal failure and oliguria to complete anuria, sometimes with malignant hypertension.

In the acute form with death in renal failure, the kidneys look normal or slightly increased in size. Sometimes there may be areas of scarring due to preexisting arterial narrowing. Petechial haemorrhages may be present. In the chronic form with a slow progression the kidneys are reduced in size.

On renal biopsy, some glomeruli may show ischaemic changes with segmental sclerosis. Others may reveal mesangial and endothelial hypercellularity and thickening of capillary tufts with tubular atrophy. Blood vessels show intimal hyperplasia.

Treatment consists of maintenance of renal perfusion and avoidance of dehydration. In the treatment of hypertension, do not cause hypotension as this will reduce renal blood flow.

RHEUMATOID ARTHRITIS

This condition has now been shown to be associated with non-specific mesangial proliferative glomerulonephritis with IgG on immunofluorescence. It is likely to be an immune complex GN.

Amyloidosis has also been associated with RA.

As a result of arteritis, some patients have a non-specific thickening of the small blood vessels in the kidneys which can lead to renal deterioration.

Chronic interstitial nephritis and papillary necrosis due to analgesics are other renal complications of the disease.

Therapy with gold and penicillamine also induces a nephrotic syndrome associated with membranous glomerulonephritis.

MULTIPLE MYELOMA

Patients affected by this condition may have nephrotic syndrome due to myeloma kidney and amyloidosis. Renal failure may be the first presenting feature of the disease. Others have the Fanconi's syndrome or nephrogenic diabetes insipidus due to hypercalcaemia.

Renal lesions of the myeloma kidney consist of tubules filled with myeloma casts surrounded by giant cells. The casts contain Bence Jones protein or amyloid. Amyloidosis and nephrocalcinosis should be looked for.

As a result of hypercalcaemia, patients may have depression, itch, constipation, thirst and confusion. Treatment of hypercalcaemia will require rehydration with saline and diuresis with frusemide. Steroids, phosphates, EDTA, mitramycin and dialysis have all been used in the treatment of hypercalcaemia.

Beware of IVP in the investigation of renal failure as it is contraindicated.

Serum electrophoresis, skeletal survey, bone marrow and renal biopsy will confirm the diagnosis.

Treatment is with steroids and cytotoxic drugs.

AMYLOIDOSIS

Nephrotic syndrome is a usual presentation. It can be due to primary amyloidosis or secondary to rheumatoid arthritis, tuberculosis, leprosy, osteomyelitis, chronic infection and myeloma.

The glomeruli show the characteristic deposits in thick lines round the blood vessels and tubules. Special staining using Congo Red and Thioflavine T will confirm amyloidosis. Electron microscopy will reveal the amyloid fibrils.

Renal vein thrombosis is a known complication in these patients.

CRYOGLOBULINAEMIA

It tends to affect females. They have arthralgia, haemolysis, Raynaud's phenomenon and nephrotic syndrome. Rheumatoid arthritis factor and anti-nuclear factor may be positive.

Some may present for the first time in chronic renal failure.

The presence of purpura and nephrotic syndrome should alert one to the possibility of the condition.

A renal biopsy will show intracapillary deposits of proteinaceous material. There is a non-specific mesangial proliferation with IgG and IgM on immunofluorescence.

MACROGLOBULINAEMIA

Males are more commonly affected. They have a bleeding tendency and purpura. Examine the fundi and look for evidence of hyperviscosity.

Treatment consists of massive fluid infusion to get rid of proteins.

A renal biopsy will show PAS deposits inside the capillaries.

RENAL TUBULAR ACIDOSIS

This has been dealt with in the chapter on Renal Tubular Acidosis.

SARCOIDOSIS

This condition is associated with direct infiltration of the kidneys causing renal failure. It also causes RTA.

Hypercalcaemia may cause the "red eye syndrome".

A chest X-ray will show enlarged lymph nodes.

Treatment consists of steroids. This will reduce the hypercalcaemia and improve renal function.

NEPHROTIC SYNDROME AND MALIGNANCY

Immune complex glomerulonephritis has been associated with cancers of the breast, colon, lymphoma and leukaemia.

Renal vein thrombosis, amyloidosis and neoplastic infiltration are often associated. Renal vein thrombosis is not a cause of nephrotic syndrome but a complication of the nephrotic syndrome.

Treatment directed at the underlying condition will result in a regression of the nephrotic syndrome.

RENAL COMPLICATIONS OF LYMPHOMA

May occur as a result of direct involvement like primary renal lymphoma, metastatic invasion of the parenchyma, hydronephrosis due to compression by lymph nodes and finally compression of the renal pedicel. All these are known causes of renal failure in this condition.

Hypercalcaemia induces nephrogenic diabetes insipidus.

Renal complications of therapy include conditions like uric acid nephropathy and radiation nephritis.

Immunological reactions may manifest as nephrotic syndrome and amyloidosis.

GOUT

See chapter on Kidney Stones.

SUBACUTE BACTERIAL ENDOCARDITIS

Renal failure is one of the causes of death in this condition. The patient presents with gross haematuria and proteinuria and casts in the urine.

Petechial haemorrhages and infarction give rise to a flea bitten kidney.

There are two types of lesions in the glomeruli:

i. Focal embolic glomerulonephritis where there are focal areas of fibrinoid necrosis or hyaline and intracapillary thrombosis.
ii. Diffuse proliferative glomerulonephritis due to an immuno-logically mediated immune complex glomerulonephritis.

One may sometimes visualise sub-epithelial humps as in post infectious glomerulonephritis. Immunofiuorescence would reveal IgG predominantly with IgA, IgM and C3.

Renal involvement takes a few weeks to develop.

XANTHOGRANULOMATOUS PYELONEPHRITIS

This is a rare condition which occurs when infection affects a kidney which is partially obstructed by calculi.

Patients with this condition have fever with chronic urinary tract infection and a mass in the loin which is seen on the

IVP as a tumour mass. Angiography however does not suggest a tumour.

Urine cultures grow *Proteus* in 60% of the cases and *E. coli* in the rest.

The gross pathology reveals large kidneys with adhesions and abscesses. Histology reveals foam cells, foreign body giant cells with necrotic debris and polymorphs. Some glomeruli will have masses of clear cells like in a carcinoma but with no mitosis. Nephrectomy may be needed if the kidney is non-functioning.

DIABETES MELLITUS

See chapter on Diabetes Mellitus.

All patients would have some degree of retinopathy with the onset of proteinuria. Other manifestations include nephrotic syndrome, hypertension, papillary necrosis and renal failure.

The glomerular lesions are:

i. Nodular Kimmelstiel-Wilson lesions which are pathognomonic of diabetic nephropathy.
ii. Diffuse intercapillary glomerulosclerosis with marked expansion of mesangial matrix. This is the commonest renal lesion for a patient with diabetic nephropathy. It is related to glomerular hyperfiltration and is accompanied by hypertrophy of the kidneys. Control of hyperglycaemia reduces hyperfiltration.
iii. Capsular drops are waxy and eosinophilic. They occur between the basement membrane and parietal epithelium of Bowman's capsule.
iv. Fibrin cap or exudate correlates with vascular disease.

Tubular lesions are Armanni-Ebstein change (glycogen nephrosis) and tubular atrophy.

Both the efferent and afferent arterioles have sub-intimal hyaline thickening due to arteriosclerosis.

The interstitium is often fibrotic with chronic inflammatory cells.

Immunofluorescence may show IgG in a linear pattern in the capillary wall. This is related to non-immunological and non-specific trapping or basement membrane dysfunction.

HENOCH~SCHONLEIN NEPHRITIS

Adults with this disease fare worse than children. There is a greater incidence of haematuria and proteinuria in adults (51%) compared to children (29%). Adults have a higher incidence of renal failure, 14% compared to 5%.

Nowadays, this condition is considered as part of the spectrum of IgA nephritis, hence the similarity in light microscopic and immunofluorescent findings with IgA nephritis.

Renal biopsy may show:

i.   Minimal lesion with a good prognosis.
ii. Focal proliferative (mesangial) GN, sometimes with sclerosis and crescents.
iii. Diffuse mesangial proliferative GN like in IgA nephritis. There may be associated sclerosis and crescents.

Immunofluorescence will show IgA predominantly with less intense staining for IgG. C3 is usually present.

The bad renal prognostic features are similar to IgA nephritis but patients with nephrotic syndrome usually do worse whatever the histology. Treatment is the same as for IgA Nephritis.

FUNCTIONAL RENAL FAILURE ASSOCIATED WITH LIVER DYSFUNCTION

The term "Hepatorenal Syndrome" is specific for renal failure which occurs secondary to liver failure due to cirrhosis of the liver. All other conditions where there is simultaneous involvement of the liver and kidneys are termed "Functional Renal Failure". These conditions include septicaemia from any cause, cholangitis, leptospirosis (which can cause renal failure because of acute tubular necrosis or interstitial nephritis), toxins (certain mushrooms) and poisons (carbon tetrachloride). Liver failure from any cause apart from cirrhosis can also cause functional renal failure.

The cause of renal failure is due to a diversion or shunting of blood to the juxta-medullary nephron with underperfusion of the cortical nephrons resulting in oliguria, low urine sodium and proximal absorption of water. This shunting could be due to failure of the liver to deconjugate vasoactive amines leading to renal shutdown. In addition, bile acids are tubulotoxic and they increase vascular sensitivity to catecholamines.

The kidneys in this condition are in fact healthy and when transplanted to healthy persons regain normal renal function.

FALCIPARUM MALARIA

Acute renal failure in this infection results from acute tubular necrosis, haemolysis, disseminated intravascular coagulation and heavy parasitic infection which causes sludging of RBC in the capillaries. Intravascular haemolysis also gives rise to haemoglobinuria.

Glomerulonephritis can also occur because of associated immunological injury. The renal biopsy would show diffuse mesangial proliferative GN with IgM, IgG and C3 on IMF. The nephritis is mild and usually resolves in 4 to 6 weeks.

Hypertension and nephrotic syndrome may also occur.

QUARTAN MALARIA

The renal manifestations may be in the form of haematuria and proteinuria, nephrotic syndrome or hypertension. In a series of 115 patients in Uganda, 26% were protein free, 45% had urinary abnorrnalities and 29% had chronic renal failure.

Renal biopsy shows focal and segmental proliferation with mesangiocapillary changes and sclerosis. IMF reveals IgG, IgM and C3 in a coarse granularity in the capillary walls.

Treatment is symptomatic, consisting of diuretics and therapy for infection and anaemia. Prednisolone, cyclophosphamide and antimalarials do not help in arresting the progression to renal failure.

REFERENCE

1. Serra A, Cameron JS, QJM, 1984, LIII, No. 210, pp 181–207.

CHAPTER 20

Pregnancy and the Kidney

Patients with most forms of kidney diseases can become pregnant. Pregnancy however may cause the kidney function to become worse in patients with glomerulonephritis if there is already mild kidney failure before pregnancy and the blood pressure proves difficult to control. In general, regardless of the type of kidney disease, as long as the patient develops hypertension in pregnancy and as long as the blood pressure is uncontrolled, the patient is at great risk of developing kidney failure. In the case of patients who already have moderate renal failure, the stress of pregnancy may cause the patient to develop end stage renal failure sometimes within a few months of pregnancy.

PRECAUTIONS DURING PREGNANCY

A patient with kidney disease who becomes pregnant will require more intensive supervision. She has to visit not only the antenatal clinic but also the renal clinic very frequently. For example, she sees the nephrologist once a month or once in two months initially, but later, she may have to report once a fortnight or even weekly, depending on the progress of the pregnancy. This is because when patients with renal disease become pregnant, especially in cases of glomerulonephritis, they run a greater risk of developing pre-eclampsia, a condition in pregnant women associated with swelling of the legs, protein loss in the urine and hypertension. Pre-eclampsia can affect the kidneys and can cause kidney failure.

Regular and frequent visits to the nephrologist allows the monitoring of renal function. Blood tests (blood urea, creatinine and uric acid) and urine examination can detect worsening renal abnormalities including the presence of excess amounts of albumin in the urine. If the patient has pre-eclampsia it may precipitate kidney failure. This is especially when it is also associated with hypertension, and most of the time it is usually the uncontrolled hypertension in a patient with kidney disease and pregnancy which causes the patient to develop kidney failure. Hence the importance of frequent follow-ups to detect early kidney failure and uncontrolled hypertension.

If renal function progressively deteriorates in pregnancy and blood pressure becomes uncontrolled, the nephrologist may have to advise the termination of pregnancy.

In many pregnant patients with kidney disease prematurity appears more common. For some mothers an early delivery may be necessary at 36 or 38 weeks. This is because in some cases the placenta cannot support the baby any longer and to persist with pregnancy may risk the health of the foetus.

PREGNANCY AND SYSTEMIC LUPUS ERYTHEMATOSUS (SLE)

This patient can become pregnant provided she has normal kidney function, blood pressure is well controlled and the disease is not active. However, she still runs the risk of developing renal failure as the disease is aggravated by pregnancy. The drugs the mother takes can also damage the foetus. (See chapter on Lupus Nephritis.)

The drugs taken by a patient with SLE are prednisolone and azathioprine. In laboratory animals these drugs cause malformation of the offspring. But in practice the risk is small, ie. 1 in 200 babies. About 25% of SLE patients who become pregnant will abort their foetus.

Immediately after pregnancy, the activity of the disease may become greater and some doctors raise the dosage of the drugs just before this stage as a precaution.

PREGNANCY IN A PATIENT ON DIALYSIS OR WITH A KIDNEY TRANSPLANT

The patient on regular dialysis can become pregnant. However, the incidence of pregnancy is low and when they do become pregnant it is important that the patient be dialysed more often in an attempt to improve the uraemic environment within the womb. The less uraemic the mother is, the better the foetus' chances of survival.

The patient who has undergone a kidney transplant can also become pregnant though the incidence is lower than in a normal woman because the prednisolone and azathioprine given to the patient may sometimes cause foetal abnormality.

PREGNANCY IN A PATIENT WITH INHERITED RENAL DISORDERS

Patients with inherited disorders will need advice before contemplating pregnancy. In the case of a pregnant patient with polycystic kidneys, there is a possibility of the enlarged kidney causing obstruction to the passage of the baby during delivery.

CHAPTER 21

Cancer and the Kidney

Cancers of the kidney are very uncommon. In fact, kidney tumours account for less than 1% of deaths from all forms of cancers.

HYPERNEPHROMA

Cancer can occur in any organ and the kidney is no exception. When it arises in the kidney it is called renal carcinoma or hypernephroma. The cancer cells are actually cells in the renal tubules which have undergone a cancerous or malignant change. It is commoner in males and the peak age is from 60 to 70 years.

The patient may have blood in the urine, pain over the side of the abdomen or he may feel a weight or a mass in the side. Sometimes he may have fever associated with loss of weight and appetite.

Investigation consists of an intravenous pyelogram (IVP), ultrasound examination and renal arteriogram. Surgical removal of the tumour is the best form of treatment especially if the tumour has not spread beyond the capsule of the kidney. Radiotherapy to the tumour bed may be of some use but treatment with drugs (chemotherapy) is of little effect.

If the tumour is confined to the kidney during operation, a 60% 5-year survival rate can be expected. The overall survival is 40% at 5 years and 25% at 10 years.

WILMS' TUMOUR

This is a malignant tumour of the kidney which occurs in childhood, usually before the age of 5 years. The child is noticed to have a swollen abdomen and examination would reveal a mass on one side of the abdomen. The child may sometimes complain of pain in the abdomen. This tumour may also be associated with fever, high blood pressure or blood in the urine.

Surgery is usually performed to remove the tumour. This is followed by radiotherapy to the tumour bed and the surrounding areas. A drug called Actinomycin D is also given to destroy tumour cells. About 80% will survive 5 years. The outlook is poorer if the tumour has already spread to other areas.

ADENOMA OF THE KIDNEY

This is a benign tumour of the kidney. It is usually diagnosed during the investigation of some other unrelated complaint and the benign tumour shows up as a distortion of the kidney, usually as an abnormality on the IVP.

CHAPTER 22

Inherited Kidney Diseases

Most forms of kidney diseases are not hereditary. Some however, can be inherited but these are rare and have a recessive pattern of inheritance. This is because in nature few individuals with dominant forms of disease would survive. Polycystic kidney disease in fact is the only common dominant form of kidney disease. It does not affect all individuals seriously and they can usually have a family.

PATTERNS OF INHERITANCE OF DISEASE

Dominant inheritance means that as long as the abnormal chromosome is passed to the offspring from one parent, the disease will appear in the offspring.

Recessive inheritance means that the individuals who carry the abnormal chromosomes are well. They are called carriers of the disease but are unaffected by it. Only if they marry another carrier will the disease appear in the offspring.

POLYCYSTIC KIDNEY

Polycystic kidney is the commonest form of inherited kidney disease. The kidneys are enlarged and replaced by cysts. Usually both kidneys are affected but one kidney may be larger than the other. It may appear at any age from infancy to old age but is usually diagnosed between 20 to 40 years.

Polycystic kidney in an individual is usually diagnosed after an affected relative has been discovered and the other family members are called up for screening. Or the patient may present with high blood pressure, blood in the urine, chronic renal failure or urinary infections, and investigations for these manifestations lead to polycystic kidneys as the cause.

The most serious problem with this disease is chronic renal failure due to progressive loss of kidney function. The kidneys are slowly replaced by the enlarging cysts, and the patient usually develops end stage renal failure between the age of 45 and 65 years.

Renal failure begins in the 3rd and 4th decade of life when the GFR begins to decrease. Evolution of chronic renal failure is homogenous within families because genetic factors contribute to determining the age of onset of uraemia. The incidence of chronic renal failure is high amongst those with hypertension. The cause of chronic renal failure is attributed to:

i. progressive arteriolar sclerosis resulting from activation of the renin angiotensin system (RAS). Patients have increased susceptibility determined by abnormal gene product and;

ii. progressive interstitial fibrosis mediated by PDGF which causes increased proliferation of fibroblasts which in time leads to progressive fibrosis of the tubulo-interstitium. Hence ADPCK is considered a chronic tubulo-interstitial nephritis. PDGF is secreted by the epithelial cell of the cyst wall.

Hypertension is the most potent predictor of renal failure in ADPCK. The hypertension is caused by:

i. impaired Sodium excretion and

ii. increased production of renin from the parenchyma adjacent to expanding cysts giving rise to Angiotensin II mediated hypertension. Even normotensive ADPCK patients have been found to have increased renin activity (high PRA) suggesting a particular role of ACE inhibitor in the management of these patients.

In hypertensive ADPCK disease, treatment with ACE inhibitor will control hypertension as well as ameliorate progressive arteriolar sclerosis resulting from activation of RAS, hence retarding progression of renal failure.

Reference:

E Ritz et al: Autosomal dominant PCK — mechanisms of cyst formation and renal failure. Aust NZ J Med, 1993; 23:35–41.

Inheritance of Polycystic Kidneys

Adult Polycystic Kidney Disease is due to an abnormal gene product on the short arm of chromosome 16.

It is inherited in a dominant pattern which means that it has the potential to appear in every successive generation. Sometimes it may skip a whole generation. About 1 in 5 patients with polycystic kidneys has no known affected relative. Children of affected parents have a 1 in 2 chance of carrying the abnormal gene. Their children have a 1 in 4 chance of getting the disease.

This condition is usually not detected on the intravenous pyelogram (IVP) until the child is about 20 years old. So an

IVP or ultrasound examination when the child is young may not detect the disease. However, even if cysts are seen, it does not mean that the child will always develop symptoms of the disease later on. A good number of people go through life without experiencing any clinical manifestations of the disease and majority do not have kidney failure. Once the disease is diagnosed the person should have an annual check of the blood pressure, and perform urine and blood tests once a year since the complications of these diseases are chronic renal failure, hypertension and urinary infections.

The brother and sister of an individual with the disease will have a 1 in 2 chance of being affected. Sometimes new patients are found to have the disease without any known family history of the disease. In these individuals, a change or mutation could have taken place causing a defect in the chromosome which gives rise to the disease.

Patients with this condition will require treatment for hypertension or urinary tract infection. Sometimes stones may form in the cysts and very rarely, a neoplastic change. Berry's aneurysm is another associated feature. Rupture of the aneurysm causes cerebral haemorrhage.

Infantile Polycystic Kidneys

Infantile polycystic kidney is another form of polycystic kidney that appears in infancy. The baby is born with enormous kidneys and dies shortly after. The disease is different from the dominant adult form of polycystic kidney as it is inherited in a recessive fashion and has a very poor outlook compared to the adult form. Parents who have an affected child have a 1 in 4 chance of having another child with the same disease in any subsequent pregnancy.

MEDULLARY SPONGE KIDNEY

This is a condition where there are many tiny ductular cysts (tubular ectasia) in the medulla or inner portion of the kidneys. The outlook for patients with this condition is very good as they do not develop kidney failure compared to polycystic kidney disease. However they are prone to two complications. One is urinary infection and the other is very small stones forming in the kidney. It is not a hereditary disorder.

INHERITED RENAL STONES

Cystinuria is a condition that is inherited in an autosomal recessive fashion. It causes recurrent kidney stones in the patient because the patient excretes excessive amounts of the amino acid cystine in the urine. Patients usually respond well to treatment with a combination of high fluid intake, alkalinisation of urine and a drug called penicillamine. If the patient can be kept free of recurrent stones he should not develop kidney failure. This will require cooperation on the part of the patient to adhere to his medical treatment.

HEREDITARY GLOMERULONEPHRITIS

Most forrns of glomerulonephritis are not hereditary. However there are a few rare forms that run in families.

1. Alport's Syndrome

This is a form of glomerulonephritis where the patient passes blood in the urine and develops progressive deafness. It is a sex-linked disorder with males more severely affected than females. When a male is affected he is usually deaf by

10 years and has chronic renal failure by 15 years. But in the case of the affected female she only has some blood and protein in the urine and is none the worse even years afterwards.

2. Benign Familial Haematuria

This is a condition where individuals in a family pass blood in the urine, usually microscopic amounts, but they do not develop deafness or renal failure.

3. Congenital Nephrotic Syndrome

The affected child is born with the condition where he has swelling of the face and limbs, passes a lot of protein in the urine and has low serum albumin level because of the protein loss in the urine. It is inherited as a recessive disease and parents have a 1 in 4 chance of further having affected children with subsequent pregnancies. It is particularly common in Finland but is very rare here.

FABRY'S DISEASE (ANGIOKERATOMA CORPORIS DIFFUSUM)

1. This is an X-linked recessive disease. It is a glycosphingolipidosis affecting young adults which leads to renal failure.
2. Manifestations include peripheral neuropathy, cutaneous nonblanching angiectases, vascular occlusions of the cardiovascular and the central nervous system. The renal lesions are characterised by fat deposits.
3. An enzyme called trihexosyl ceramidase is deficient and this leads to deposition of fat in the tissues.

4. The patient requires a renal transplant to cure the condition as the donor kidney produces the deficient enzyme.

CONGENITAL MALFORMATION AND DEVELOPMENTAL ANOMALIES

These include horseshoe kidneys, duplex kidneys (duplication of the kidneys or the pelvis and ureter), bifid ureter and other malformations like agenesis and hypoplastic kidney as well as cysts, aberrant renal arteries and retrocaval ureter.

CHAPTER 23

Drugs and the Kidney

In a patient with renal impairment it is necessary to adjust the dose or the dosing interval of certain drugs which are excreted by the kidneys. Drugs which are excreted by the kidneys are water soluble. Lipophilic drugs are metabolised in the liver into water soluble metabolites before excretion by the kidneys. Apart from the excretion of the drug itself, one has also to consider the elimination of metabolites which may still possess significant pharmacological properties like cyclosporin A and its toxic metabolites.

In clinical practice, one generally administers an initial dose and the maintenance doses are reduced according to the degree of renal failure using various formulae based on the weight of the patient and the level of the serum creatinine.

For example: If one wants to prescribe gentamicin to a male patient weighing 60 kg with a serum creatinine of 3.2 mg/dl:

The loading dose would be 1 mg/kg BW which would be 60 mg of gentamicin.

The dosing interval in hours would be: Serum creatinine multiplied by a factor of 7, ie. $3.2 \times 7 = 22.4$ hours or once a day dosing interval. The next dosing interval would depend on the next day's serum creatinine level. One could increase the dose and prolong the dosing interval or reduce the dose and shorten the dosing interval.

For amikacin, a factor of 9 is used in the calculation.

The above calculation at best is still a very crude approximation as too many assumptions have been made. In practice, blood for the estimation of gentamicin or amikacin levels, both peak and trough levels, would have been sent off and the subsequent doses would be deterrnined by these levels.

THE EFFECTS OF DRUGS ON THE KIDNEYS

I. Renal Haemodynamic Changes

1 . NSAID or non-steroidal anti-inflammatory drugs like indomethacin, naprosyn and mefenamic acid decrease GFR. They inhibit the synthesis of prostaglandins since they are prostaglandin synthetase inhibitors and prostaglandins are important in maintaining vasodilation and promotion of renal blood flow.

2. ACEI and ATRA like enalapril and losartan can cause renal failure because they antagonise the angiotensin II receptors at the efferent arterioles of glomeruli, and thereby decrease intraglomerular BP resulting in lowered GFR.

3. Cyclosporin A can cause severe tubulo-interstitial injury as well as inhibition of prostaglandin synthesis resulting in renal failure. (See chapter on Renal Transplantation.) Cyclosporin A also causes increased platelet aggregation and predisposes to thrombosis of renal blood vessels.

II. Direct Tubular Toxicity

1 . Lithium carbonate is toxic to the distal tubules and causes nephrogenic diabetes insipidus.

2. Amphotericin B produces tubular damage with renal impairment. It also causes Distal or Type I RTA.
3. Outdated tetracyclines cause Fanconi's syndrome (Type II RTA). Tetracycline too causes a hypercatabolic state with marked elevation of blood urea in patients with renal impairment.
4. Analgesics like aspirin, even paracetamol in high doses and NSAID cause papillary necrosis of the kidneys (analgesic nephropathy).
5. Aminoglycosides damage predominantly the proximal tubules.

Characteristically they produce non-oliguric acute renal failure. This occurs more commonly in the elderly, especially when they are dehydrated or given diuretics. Combination with cephaloridine further aggravates the nephrotoxicity. The second and third generation cephalosporins do not have a synergistic nephrotoxic effect with the aminoglycosides.

III. Blockage of Renal Tubules

1. Sulphonamides can cause crystalluria because of poor solubility especially in an acidic urine. It is therefore important to alkalinise the urine of patients who are prescribed sulphonamides.
2. Methotrexate in high dose can cause acute tubular necrosis due to its precipitation in the renal tubules.
3. Methoxyflurane causes oxaluria with intratubular precipitation of calcium oxalate crystals, giving rise to renal failure.
4. Triamterene (see chapter on Diuretics) can cause crystals and casts to form in the tubules, giving rise to triamterene stones.

IV. Immunologically Mediated Damage

1. Sulphonamides, bactrium, allopurinol, methicillin, even ampicillin can all cause an acute allergic interstitial nephritis associated with Steven Johnson's syndrome. See chapter on Renal Tubular Disorders.
2. Penicillamine produces a membranous glomerulonephritis resulting in the nephrotic syndrome.
3. Rifampicin can give rise to an immune complex glomerulonephritis and methicillin can cause a rapidly progressive glomerulonephritis due to formation of anti-glomerular basement membrane antibodies (anti-GBM antibodies).

V. Injury Related to Changes in Electrolytes

1. Diuretics can cause hypokalaemia inducing vacuolar degeneration of the tubules with nephrogenic diabetes insipidus.
2. Vitamin D therapy can induce hypercalcaemia predisposing to intrarenal calcification and tubular damage with renal impairment.

PRACTICE POINTS

1. In any patient with renal impairment it is always useful to take a drug history, especially with regard to the use of analgesics both from the point of analgesic nephropathy as well as NSAID related renal failure. Remember that ACE inhibitors prescribed for hypertension can also cause renal impairment.
2. In a patient with rash and renal impairment, think of acute allergic interstitial nephritis. Enquire about the use of allopurinol, bactrium and other antibiotics given by other

doctors. Check for eosinophilia and eosinophils in the urine.

3. Remember aminoglycosides as a very common cause of renal impairment when dealing with a patient who has sepsis and renal failure. Check the levels of aminoglycosides in the serum.

4. Withdrawal of the offending agent, eg. ACE inhibitor will result in an improvement of renal function.

5. Sometimes a renal biopsy may have to be performed to confirm or exclude acute interstitial nephritis.

DRUGS WHICH REQUIRE CAUTION AND ALTERATION OF DOSAGE IN RENAL FAILURE

A 1. Antibiotics

• Aminoglycosides: Marked decrease in dose required. Monitor drug levels.

• Cephalosporins: Avoid cephaloridine which is very nephrotoxic. The newer generation may require some alteration of dosage.

• Ciprofloxacin: Adjust dose when large doses are used.

• Nitrofurantoin: Avoid in renal failure since it causes very painful neuropathy. Like nalidixic acid it is also useless in renal failure as both are not concentrated in the kidneys in renal failure to be of any use.

• Penicillin: Adjust dose only when large doses are used.

• Tetracycline: Avoid in renal failure because of catabolic effect. Doxycycline can be used.

• Acyclovir, Ganciclovir: Reduce dose; can cause mild renal impairment.

- Amphotericin B: Slight reduction in dose. Usually causes renal impairment even in patients with normal renal function.

- Bactrium or Septrin (combination of sulphonamide and trimethoprim): Adjust dose in renal failure.

- Ethambutol: Reduce dose.

- 5-fluorocytosine: Marked decrease in dose.

- Isoniazid: Reduce in advanced renal failure.

- Para-amino-salicylic acid: Avoid in renal failure.

- Streptomycin: Marked reduction of dose.

A 2. Anti-Convulsants

- Phenobarb: Reduce dose in advanced renal failure.

- Phenytoin: Reduce dose in advanced renal failure.

A 3. Anticoagulants and Anti-Platelet Agents

- Warfarin, heparin and dipyridamole: May be useful to reduce dose as patients with renal failure have a tendency to bleed. Use of these agents withdrawn when Serum Creatinine exceeds 500 micro M/L.

A 4. Antineoplastic agents

- Cisplatin
  Primary site of nephrotoxicity is at distal tubular and collecting ducts.
  Use with moderate hydration (3 litres per day) and mannitol or frusemide diuresis to reduce nephrotoxicity

Do not exceed 120 mg/M^2 body surface area as it causes irreversible toxicity.

• Nephrotoxicity due to these agents can be manifest as acute renal failure, chronic renal failure or specific tubular dysfunction.

C. Cardiac Drugs

• Digoxin: Marked reduction in dose.

D. Diuretics

• Frusemide and other loop diuretics: Require large doses to be effective.
Burinex more effective (1 mg ≡ 40 mg of Frusemide). Beware of dehydration and aggravation of renal failure.

• Spironolactone: Avoid in renal failure as it is a potassium sparing diuretic.

• Thiazides: Not effective in renal failure.

H 1. H 2 Antagonists

• Cimetidine, ranitidine: Reduce dose; ranitidine is preferred.

H 2. Hypolipidaemic Drugs

• Eicosapentanoic acid: Caution, reduce dose because of bleeding tendency in uraemics.

• Gemfibrozil: Caution, reduce dose in renal failure.
Simvastatin, Pravastatin : In severe renal failure, reduce dose.

- Never combine Gemfibrozil and statin as this will cause myoglobinuria with renal failure.

H 3. Hypotensive Drugs

- ACE inhibitors: Reduce dose in renal failure, monitor renal function and serum potassium. *ACE inhibitor and Angiotensin Receptor Antagonist (ATRA) used to reduce intra-glomerular hypertension in patients with glomerular hyperfiltration. Withdraw when Serum Creatinine exceeds 500 micro M/L as danger of hyperkalaemia increased.

- Beta blockers: Reduce dose as metabolites are active (Atenolol).

I. Immunosuppressive Drugs

- Azathioprine: Reduce dose.

- Cyclophosphamide: Reduce dose.

- Cyclosporin A: Reduce dose, monitor levels.

N. Non-Steroidal Anti-Inflammatory Drugs (NSAID)

- Aspirin, indocid, ponstan, naproxen, ketoprofen, diclofenac, sulindac, vioxx, celebrex (celecoxib, cycloxygenese-L-inhibitors): Try to avoid as they can cause or worsen renal failure.

  Codeine or Gingerol (Zinax) may be useful substitutes as analgesics.
  Gingerol is mild and slow acting.

O. Oral Hypoglycaemics

- Avoid long acting oral hypoglycemics like Chlorpropamide, Glibenclamide in renal failure. Use short acting ones like Tolbutamide and Diamicron (Gliclazide) and short to intermediate acting ones like Minidiab (Glipizide).

- Metformin: Avoid in renal failure as there is risk of lactic acidosis. Avoid in patients with diabetic nephropathy.

Renal Transplant: Drugs to avoid

- Allopurinol: Avoid in a transplant patient on Azathioprine. It interferes with metabolism of Azathioprine through purine pathway as it is a xanthine oxidase inhibitor, thus potentiating effect of Azathioprine and causing bone marrow suppression.

- Erythromycin: Caution in transplant patient on Cyclosporine A. Avoid if possible. Will cause CyA toxicity as it interferes with liver enzyme (Cytochrome P 450) which metabolises CyA. Check CyA levels and reduce dose of CyA.

CHAPTER 24

Acute Renal Failure

DEFINITION

Acute renal failure is a sudden temporary and usually "reversible" failure of the kidneys to excrete waste products of metabolism. The first sign is oliguria, usually defined as urine volume less than 400 ml per day. In addition to traditionally described oliguric acute renal failure, there is non-oliguric acute renal failure which is also transient and reversible where the urine output is about a litre or more. Here there is less morbidity and mortality compared to oliguric renal failure. Non-oliguric renal failure is often caused by nephrotoxic antibiotics (in particular the aminoglycosides) and anaesthetics.

DIAGNOSTIC APPROACH AND INVESTIGATION

In the history one should always enquire about recent surgery, trauma, hypertension, drugs and previous renal diseases.

In the physical examination pay attention to the state of hydration of the patient whether he is dehydrated or in fluid overload (presence of oedema, jugular venous pressure (JVP), postural hypotension), external genitalia, palpation of the kidneys, urinary bladder, rectal and vaginal examination.

Establish whether patient is in "pre-renal" (hypovolaemia), "renal", or post-renal" (urinary obstruction) failure.

Exclude Obstruction (Post Renal Failure)

In the history, enquire about renal calculi, prostatic symptoms, recent surgery, trauma to pelvis and cancer.

On examination look for a full urinary bladder or full and tender loin. An ultrasound of the kidneys, CT scan or cystoscopy and retrograde pyelogram may be necessary.

Once obstruction has been excluded, decide whether patient has "prerenal failure" (hypotension, dehydration, hypovolaemia, hypoperfusion) or "intrinsic renal failure" due to an intrinsic renal cause (acute tubular necrosis or vasomotor nephropathy).

INVESTIGATIONS

1. In "pre-renal failure" (hypovolaemia), the urine microscopy is normal but in vasomotor nephropathy (acute tubular necrosis) the urine contains some protein, tubular cells and casts.
2. If RBC casts are present in the urine the patient is likely to have glomerulonephritis as the cause of renal failure rather than vasomotor nephropathy or acute tubular necrosis.
3. If total urinary protein exceeds 2 gm, the diagnosis favours a chronic nephritis rather than vasomotor nephropathy.
4. Eosinophils in the urine should alert one to the possibility of allergic interstitial nephritis.
5. If the patient has total or absolute anuria and obstruction has been excluded, then a diagnosis of occlusion of the renal arteries has to be considered.
6. As and when appropriate, one may have to request for an ultrasound examination of the kidneys, a CT scan or renal arteriogram.

A high dose intravenous pyelogram may reveal the following:
1. Small smooth shrunken kidneys which would suggest chronic glomerulonephritis.
2. Small scarred kidneys which may suggest pyelonephritis (reflux nephropathy), diabetic nephropathy, analgesic nephropathy or even renal artery stenosis.
3. Total absence of the nephrogram phase would suggest arterial occlusion or a severe proliferative glomerulonephritis.
4. Early dense persisting nephrogram may favour vasomotor nephropathy or acute suppurative pyelonephritis.
5. A slowly developing dense nephrogram suggests acute glomerulonephritis.
6. A faintly persistent nephrogram suggests a chronic glomerulonephritis.

High dose IVP is not done nowadays because of contrast media induced nephrotoxicity.

INTRINSIC RENAL FAILURE

The following are some of the possibilities:
1. Vasomotor nephropathy (VMN) or acute tubular necrosis (ATN)
2. Glomerulonephritis, vasculitis
3. Acute interstitial nephritis, drugs
4. Renal vascular thrombosis
5. Acute exacerbation of chronic glomerulonephritis

1. Vasomotor Nephropathy or Acute Tubular Necrosis

The term vasomotor nephropathy is now preferred to the traditional term acute tubular necrosis as it has now been shown that patients with ATN or VMN have vasoconstriction of the afferent arteriole. In many cases diagnosed clinically as acute tubular necrosis, the renal biopsies often show normal histology except for some mild vacuolar degeneration even though patients behave like classical ATN clinically.

Recognise the precipitating causes like shock, haemorrhage, dehydration, septicaemia and leptospirosis. There should be absence of evidence suggesting preexisting acute or chronic renal disease, allergic interstitial nephritis or vascular occlusion.

2. Glomerulonephritis, Vasculitis

Most patients in this category would give a history suggesting acute glomerulonephritis or a systemic illness like systemic lupus erythematosus.

If the urine microscopy demonstrates RBC casts, glomerulonephritis as a cause of renal failure is likely.

A total urinary proteinuria exceeding 2 gm suggests glomerulonephritis.

Low serum complement would indicate glomerulonephritis or SLE. A high ESR, positive LE cell, positive ANF and positive anti-DNA would point to SLE.

Renal biopsy may show post infectious glomerulonephritis, crescenteric glomerulonephritis, lupus nephritis, polyarteritis nodosa.

3. Interstitial Nephritis, Drugs

Allergic interstitial nephritis presents with fever, rash, eosinophilia and eosinophils in the urine. A renal biopsy readily confirms the diagnosis through the presence of widespread tubulo-interstitial nephritis with plentiful cellular infiltrates including eosinophils. This condition should be treated with prednisolone to prevent interstitial scarring and promote rapid healing and reversal of the allergic phenomenon. Methicillin, sulphonamides and allopurinol have all been implicated.

Contrast media used in radiology, antibiotics (gentamicin, amikacin, cephalosporin, streptomycin), and diuretics (thiazides) may also be responsible.

In Singapore, leptospirosis is a common cause of acute interstitial nephritis causing acute renal failure. The serum erythrocyte lysis (SEL) test should always be performed in any patient presenting with systemic infection and renal failure.

Other causes of interstitial nephritis are toxins from bee stings and other insects, and venoms from snake bites.

4. Renal Vascular (Arterial Thrombosis, Embolism)

While taking a history, enquire regarding possibility of subacute bacteria endocarditis and mural thrombi. Loin pain and hypertension associated with oligo-anuria may suggest renal infarction.

Absent nephrogram on intravenous pyelogram or a renal radioisotope scan or a renal arteriogram showing no blood flow would indicate renal vascular obstruction.

Renal artery thrombosis may follow trauma or it could result from atherosclerosis. The patient would require urgent endarterectomy.

5. Acute Exacerbation of Chronic Renal Disease

The patient may reveal a history of previous symptoms of renal impairment, hypertension or urinary tract infection.

Urine microscopy may show RBC, casts, or protein. The total urinary protein usually ranges from 1 to 2 gm/day in these cases. A renal biopsy would confirm the diagnosis of preexisting glomerulonephritis.

In patients with "acute on chronic" renal failure, the acute elements causing acute renal failure may be dehydration, sepsis, uncontrolled hypertension, obstruction and nephrotoxic antibiotics as well as contrast agents and NSAIDS. When considering obstruction one should exclude obstruction to the urological tract as well as thrombosis of renal veins and arteries.

Tables 24.1 and 24.2 show the causes of acute renal failure in Singapore.

Table 24.1 Causes of acute renal failure in Singapore (1976–1982)

	No. of Cases	%
1. Infection	28	30%
2. Glomerulonephritis	9	10%
3. Renal Stone	6	7%
4. Drugs	7	8%
5. Poisoning	12	13%
6. Pregnancy Related	8	8%
7. Hepato-renal Failure	6	7%
8. Post Surgery	9	10%
9. Cancer	4	4%
10. Others	3	3%
TOTAL	92	100%

+ Table 24.2   Causes of acute renal failure in Singapore (1985–1989)

Causes	No. of Patients	No. of Death
1. Septicaemia	23	12
2. Glomerulonephritis	3	1
3. Hepatorenal Syndrome	1	1
4. Drugs	2	0
5. Poisoning	2	1
6. Malignancy	1	1
7. Renal stone	2	1
8. Ruptured Viscus	2	2
9. Trauma	4	2
10. Miscellaneous*	8	4
TOTAL	48	25 (52%)

Acute Myocardial Infarction, Pancreatitis, Rhabdomyolysis, Hornet sting.
+ *Courtesy of S S Wei.*

CLINICAL COURSE OF ACUTE RENAL FAILURE

I. Onset Phase

Often the problem is one of diagnosis at onset rather than problem of immediate treatment. At this stage the patient has few symptoms or signs of renal failure other than oliguria. There is mild elevation of blood urea and serum creatinine and deteriorating electrolyte disturbance.

II. Oliguric Phase

In the majority of patients, there is often fluid overload with hyponatraemia associated with ankle oedema and pulmonary oedema. A routine chest X-ray should be performed in all patients.

If the patient has hyponatraemia it is important to exclude depletional hyponatraemia due to dehydration or gastrointestinal loss due to vomiting.

Hyperkalaemia is often due to oliguria, release of K^+ from cells as a result of trauma, haemolysis, catabolism, infection or acidosis. Symptoms of hyperkalaemia may manifest as paresthesia, weakness of muscles and cardiac arrhythmias.

Acidosis occurs because the damaged kidneys cannot excrete H^+, hence the Kussmaul's respiration.

Acute Uraemic Syndrome

The acute uraemic syndrome is due to uraemic toxins affecting the cardiovascular, gastrointestinal, central nervous and the haematological systems.

Cardiovascular system: Patients may present with hypertension, arrhythmias, congestive heart failure and pericardititis.

Gastrointestinal: Anorexia, nausea, vomiting, diarrhoea, gastrointestinal bleeding (gastric erosion, colitis, oesophagitis) and pancreatitis.

Central nervous system: Confusion, twitching, asterixis and fits due to uraemic encephalopathy may be present.

Haemopoietic system: The anaemia of renal failure is a normochromic, normocytic anaemia. It is caused by decreased erythropoietin. Sometimes, depending on the cause of renal failure, haemolysis or blood loss may contribute to the anaemia. Platelet function may be abnormal. This takes the form of decreased platelet adhesiveness and decreased platelet aggregation.

The patient with renal failure is also prone to pneumonia, urinary infections, skin infections and decreased wound healing as he has decreased phagocytosis and immune paralysis due to the depression of the immune system by the uraemic environment.

III. Diuretic Phase

Restoration of renal function is heralded by the diuretic phase. The onset of this phase is unpredictable and may occur anytime from 24 hours to even 2 months. It is related to the removal of excess water and salt as well as to impaired renal concentration. The danger to the patient at this stage is excess loss of water, dehydration and hypokalaemia. During this time patients experience a sense of well-being. There is loss of nausea and the appetite returns.

MANAGEMENT OF ACUTE RENAL FAILURE

I. Oliguric Phase

At this stage one strives to keep the patient alive until his kidneys undergo a cure. It is important to monitor the electrolytes as well as the blood urea and serum creatinine daily. Maintain an intake and output chart. When the patient is oliguric his fluid intake should not exceed 500 ml/day unless he is dehydrated. Usually, patients tend to be overloaded as they are not passing into the urine the amount of water they have been drinking.

Serum potassium especially has to be monitored from the daily electrolyte profile. Hyperkalaemia (serum $K^+ >$ 6 mEq/l) should be treated. An injection of 12 units of soluble insulin together with 50 ml of 50% dextrose is given in a bolus dose or in a drip infusion over half to 1 hour. If the patient can take orally, commence Resonium A 15 gm 8 hourly. If the patient cannot take orally, commence Resonium retention enema 30 gm 8-hourly. Also administer I.V. calcium gluconate or chloride 10 ml slowly to combat the effects of hyperkalaemia on the heart. Repeat serum K^+ 4 hours later and if serum K^+ proves difficult to control, dialysis may be required or a second bolus of insulin and dextrose may be given.

The caloric intake of the patient must be adequate to prevent catabolism of the body proteins. Anaemia is corrected by transfusion of packed red blood cells. Hypertension and heart failure should be treated. Infections should be treated with the correct antibiotics. The choice of antibiotics and the dosage is important. The use of aminoglycosides should be monitored by drug levels (gentamicin or amikacin levels).

If necessary the patient should be dialysed. The patient should be dialysed when serum creatinine is about 700 micro mol/L (sometimes even earlier). Other indications for dialysis are uraemic symptoms, pericarditis, hyperkalaemia, severe acidosis, pulmonary oedema or a hypercatabolic state. In patients with unstable BP, continuous renal replacement therapy (CRRT) like hemofiltration or hemodialfiltration is performed.

II. Diuretic Phase

The hazard at this stage is excessive loss of fluid, Na^+ and K^+. The high urea content in blood induces an osmotic diuresis. In addition, a defect in tubular concentration due to ATN is another cause for the diuretic phase. Sometimes efforts to keep up with the diuresis may perpetuate it.

One should maintain a strict intake and output chart. Check urine volume, serum urea, creatinine and electrolytes. Fluids and K^+ should be replaced accordingly.

III. Post Diuretic Phase

The urine output of the patient slowly normalises as the renal blood flow and GFR gradually increase. Tubular functions like concentration and dilution may take a longer time to recover.

PROGNOSIS

Recovery depends on the nature of the underlying disease, ie. the cause of renal failure. 50% of hospital acquired acute renal failure are multifactoial. Patients with trauma, infection and shock do worse. A healthy young patient does better than an old patient.

Efficient management is also important in determining prognosis. The mortality rate is now about 37% in non intensive care unit (ICU) patients. For simple acute renal failure patients, with no other illness, outside ICU, mortality rate is 7–23%. Mortality in ICU patients is 50–80%. Survival depends on severity of underlying illness and number of failed organs, that is, co-morbid illness.

20% of all deaths are due to infections and in 60%, infections are contributory factors.

Reference: Treatment of Acute Renal Failure: Robert A. Star. Kidney International, 1998, Vol 54: 1817–1831.

CHAPTER 25

Chronic Renal Failure

DEFINITION

Chronic renal failure is the gradual onset of an "irreversible" and persistent impairment of both glomerular and tubular functions which is so severe that the kidneys are no longer able to maintain the normal internal environment. This definition includes mild asymptomatic functional impairment, sometimes called chronic renal impairment.

AETIOLOGY

1. **Primary glomerular disease:** Acute glomerular disease including rapidly progressive glomerulonephritis. Chronic glomerulonephritis is the second commonest cause of ESRF in Singapore.
2. **Primary tubular disease:** Chronic hypercalcaemia, chronic hypokalaemia, heavy metal poisoning like lead and cadmium.
3. **Vascular disease:** Ischaemia of the kidneys due to congenital or acquired renal artery stenosis; accelerated or malignant hypertension, hypertensive nephrosclerosis.
4. **Infection:** Chronic atrophic pyelonephritis (reflux nephropathy), tuberculosis.
5. **Obstruction:** Renal stones, retroperitoneal fibrosis, prostatomegaly, urethral strictures and tumours.
6. **Vasculitis:** Systemic lupus erythematosus, polyarteritis nodosa, Henoch-Schonlein nephritis, scleroderma, Wegener's

granulomatosis. In Systemic Vasculitis, anti-neutrophilic cytoplasmic antibody (ANCA) is usually positive, while it is usually negative in SLE.

7. **Metabolic renal disease:** Diabetes mellitus (commonest cause of ESRF), amyloidosis, analgesic nephropathy, gout, primary hyperparathyroidism and milk alkali syndrome.

8. **Congenital abnormality:** Hypoplastic kidneys, reflux nephropathy, medullary cystic disease, polycystic kidneys.

Every year in Singapore, about 650 patients or 163 per million population, would be in end stage renal failure.

Table 25.1 lists the causes of chronic renal failure in Singapore.

Table 25.1 Causes of chronic renal failure in Singapore. About 500 new ESRF patients are seen every year

	%
1. Diabetic Nephropathy	47%
2. Chronic Glomerulonephritis	29%
3. Hypertensive Nephrosclerosis	9%
4. Polycystic Kidney	3%
5. Vasculitis	2%
6. Kidney Stones	1%
7. Chronic Pyelonephritis	1%
8. Causes Unknown	8%
TOTAL	100%

CLINICAL PRESENTATION

Central Nervous System

One of the most subtle changes in uraemia is a neuro-behavioural change. It may take the form of a personality defect. The patient tends to speak in short sentences. He has a short attention span and performs mental arithmetic poorly. Later he becomes disorientated and then develops delirium, fits and lapses into a coma. The electroencephalogram shows slow waves indicative of a metabolic encephalopathy. Physical examination would reveal asterixis.

The peripheral nervous system is also involved and neuropathy may take the form of the restless leg syndrome, burning feet syndrome or even foot drop due to paralysis.

The urinary bladder may show a large residual volume due to an autonomic neuropathy.

Myopathy may be an added feature of the uraemic syndrome.

Patients are also prone to cerebrovascular accidents in the form of cerebral thrombosis, embolism or haemorrhage as they have accelerated atherogenesis.

Ophthalmic Changes

Acute visual loss due to cortical blindness may be a manifestation of uraemia.

Patients may have calcium deposits in the cornea (band keratopathy) due to metastatic calcification causing a red eye syndrome or "conjunctivitis".

There may be amino acid deposits in the lateral aspects of the cornea giving rise to wedge-shaped "penguinculae".

Examination of the fundi may show changes of a hypertensive fundus. One may see papilloedema due to accelerated or malignant hypertension. The finding of a macular star in the fundus should alert one to the possibility of chronic renal failure.

Gastrointestinal

Nausea and vomiting are the classical features of the uraemic syndrome. This is due to the decomposition of urea to ammonia by gastrointestinal flora which causes irritation of the gastrointestinal tract. Acute gastric erosions may cause haematemesis and melaena. Gastrointestinal bleeding may also be due to uraemic colitis which may cause diarrhoea or lower intestinal bleeding. Other gastrointestinal manifestations of uraemia include hiccups, parotitis and sometimes pancreatitis.

Dermatological

Uraemic itch is commonly due to the dry and scaly skin in uraemic patients because of atrophy of the sweat glands causing decreased sweating. Other causes of the uraemic itch include hypercalcaemia resulting from tertiary hyperparathyroidism, and peripheral neuropathy. Uraemic frost is seldom seen nowadays. This is the result of precipitation of uraemic crystals in the skin. Improved standard of hygiene and nursing care may account for the rarity of uraemic frost.

The brown nail arc is another cutaneous feature. This is due to deposits of lipochrome and urochrome in the outer edges of the nails.

Due to severe itch patients tend to scratch their skin and platelet dysfunction and capillary fragility in these patients would contribute to easy bruising seen together with the scratch marks on the skin.

The skin of the uraemic patient is also prone to bacterial, viral and fungal infections as they have decreased cell mediated immune function.

Cardiovascular System

Congestive cardiac failure may be due to severe anaemia or severe hypertension or a combination of uncontrolled hypertension with fluid overload.

Uraemic pericarditis may be a cause of chest pain. When the pain disappears it may mean that the patient has now developed pericardial effusion. The development of pericardial tamponade is always a potential danger in anyone with an effusion. This is especially so in patients who are on regular haemodialysis where heparin is routinely used. Such patients may require pericardial tapping when there is a moderate pericardial effusion.

Uncontrolled hypertension may give rise to acute left ventricular failure with paroxysmal nocturnal dyspnoea due to acute pulmonary oedema. Severe fluid overload per se is another cause of pulmonary oedema. This is contributed to by increased capillary permeability and the chest X-ray occasionally shows the classical appearance of batwings, sometimes termed uraemic lung due to pulmonary oedema.

Haematological System

The anaemia of chronic renal failure is a normochromic normocytic anaemia. This is due to decreased erythropoietin production because of uraemia. Patients may sometimes have folate deficiency as evidenced by hypersegmented polymorphonuclear leukocytes. The red blood cells in a uraemic environment have a shortened lifespan because of the uraemic toxin. The bleeding tendency associated with renal failure is the result of impaired platelet function in the form of decreased platelet adhesion and aggregation.

Respiratory System

A deep sighing respiration due to severe metabolic acidosis called Kussmaul's breathing is often seen in the patient with uraemia. Pulmonary oedema is another cause of severe dyspnoea and a chest X-ray may show the typical batwing appearance over both lung fields.

Patients with uraemia are also prone to pneumonia because of decreased resistance to infection as they have impaired cell mediated immunity as well as decreased phagocytosis in the leukocyte.

Renal Osteodystrophy

This is another term for renal bone disease which in clinical practice usually implies a combination of osteomalacia and secondary hyperparathyroidism. It is the result of impaired calcium and vitamin D metabolism. In renal failure the renal tubules are unable to convert 25-dihydroxycholecalciferol to 1,25-dihydroxycholecalciferol. This leads to decreased absorption of calcium from the bowels which in turn stimulates the parathyroid gland to secrete more parathormone. The stimulated parathyroid gland undergoes hypertrophy giving rise to secondary hyperparathyroidism where the patient has low serum calcium and high serum phosphate, and increased serum alkaline phosphatase levels. Persistent hypercalcaemia is a feature of tertiary hyperparathyroidism when the glands have become autonomous.

If the skeleton can respond to excess parathormone the patient has osteitis fibrosa cystica and if the calcium phosphate product exceeds 70 (in mg) or 6 (in S.I. units), metastatic or ectopic calcification results. The patient then has calcium deposited in the cornea of the eyes and presents with the red eye syndrome or he has band keratopathy. Metastatic calcification may also involve the joints and soft tissues of the body including various organs. Deposition in the skin causes severe pruritus while deposition in the blood vessels can make subsequent renal transplant very difficult technically.

If the skeleton cannot respond to excess parathormone then osteomalacia or adult rickets is the result.

The patient with renal osteodystrophy may present with a waddling gait or he may walk with a limp and complain of bone pain or chest pain because of fracture of the ribs. Pain in the hip may be the result of fracture of the neck of the femur.

MANAGEMENT

Search for reversible treatable chronic diseases of the kidney and treat them as this may arrest or slow down the progression of renal deterioration. In this respect, infections like renal tuberculosis and chronic pyelonephritis (reflux nephropathy) are noteworthy. The course of analgesic nephropathy can also be arrested if the patient can be made to stop the abuse of analgesics. Hypercalcaemic nephropathy, hypokalaemic nephropathy and renal disease due to drugs and chemicals should also be identified and treated. Finally, obstructive uropathy due to stones and enlarged prostate can be treated.

Look for reversible factors adversely affecting the course of irreversible renal disease, among which are causes such as urinary and any other forms of sepsis that could cause renal impairment. Dehydration or salt depletion, evident by the presence of postural hypotension, loss of tissue turgor, decreased JVP, low serum sodium and chloride can also be easily identified and treated. Hypokalaemia and heart failure are also reversible causes of renal impairment. Uncontrolled or accelerated hypertension from whatever cause also needs to be treated aggressively. Finally, nephrotoxic agents, in particular the aminoglycosides, cephalosporins, bactrium, tetracycline, allopurinol, NSAID and many others should be thought of in a patient with renal failure. Drugs and antibiotics can give rise to renal impairment either because of a direct nephrotoxic effect or due to a hypersensitivity reaction giving rise sometimes to unsuspected interstitial nephritis.

Always exclude Dehydration, Sepsis, uncontrolled Hypertension, Obstruction (to urological tract or renal vessels — thrombosis of veins or arteries) and Drugs including nephrotoxic antibiotics and NSAIDS.

Dietary Treatment

Low Protein Diet

Restriction of dietary protein relieves symptoms of uraemia like nausea and vomiting but imposition of an unpalatable diet is not an easy task and may sometimes be considered unkind. The first problem is to get the patient to take the low protein diet. The second is to persuade him to continue it.

Traditionally it has been taught that low protein diet will not prevent the progression of underlying renal disease, and often there is a decrease in the level of blood urea but serum creatinine remains the same or worsens. The diet serves to prevent the accumulation of potentially toxic metabolites and relieves symptoms of uraemia but nutrition suffers eventually.

The aim of imposing a low protein diet in a patient with renal failure therefore is to cause a decrease in the metabolic end products of nitrogen metabolism which accumulates in his body.

20 gm Protein Diet

The 20 gm protein diet contains only 3 gm of nitrogen which is the smallest quantity of nitrogen required to maintain nitrogen balance in most uraemics, though in most patients it often leads to malnourishment.

Giovanetti and Giordano introduced essential amino acids into the 20 gm low protein diet which was supplemented with higher calories. They obtained much better results as evident by a more dramatic lowering of blood urea, and in a substantial number of their patients there was also improvement or stabilisation of serum creatinine levels. Nowadays a 20 gm protein diet is not prescribed as it is considered a starvation diet.

0.8 gm/kg BW Protein Diet

Most individuals require at least 35 gm (0.5 gm/kg BW) of protein in order to maintain nitrogen balance reasonably well. At the Singapore General Hospital, a low protein diet usually means a 0.8 gm/kg BW protein diet. Therefore a 50 kg weight patient would require a 40 gm protein diet and a 60 kg weight patient a 50 gm protein diet. It is important to stress that patients on low protein diet require not only high biological protein with essential amino acids but also high calorie carbohydrate and fat.

Excellent nutritional care may minimise complications such as malaise, nausea, vomiting, haemorrhage, anaemia, osteodystrophy, neuropathy, infections, and psychological problems.

Hyperfiltration and Relevance of Low Protein Diet (0.8 gm/kg BW)

Nowadays most nephrologists believe that in today's setting, protein restriction should be commenced when the serum creatinine is above normal (> 141 micro mol/L or > 1.5 mg/dl) as it is thought that early protein restriction in patients with mild renal impairment may decrease the damage due to glomerular hyperfiltration. Protein restriction is not necessary once serum creatinine is above 500 micro mol/L. Patients should have a normal protein diet at this stage. Otherwise the patient may have malnutrition by the time he needs dialysis.

Keto Acid Analogues

Keto and hydroxy analogues of the amino acids have been much popularised. These agents are transaminated in the liver by non-essential amino acids to the corresponding essential amino acids which are then used for protein synthesis. 20 gm high biological value protein diets supplemented with keto acid analogues in patients with creatinine clearance of less than 15 ml/min have resulted in slowing and even temporarily reversing the progression of chronic renal failure. Compliance may be a problem in these patients as it involves a Giovanetti type high biological value diet together with keto acid analogue supplements. The practical role of these agents may be restricted to patients for whom dialysis is not readily available.

Maintaining Internal Environment

In the management of patients with chronic renal failure one should try to maintain the internal environment as near normal as possible.

Prevent dehydration and salt depletion as well as fluid overload. Examine the patient and monitor the neck veins, tissue turgor and tongue. Check the blood pressure for postural hypotension and the serum electrolytes. The patient may require salt supplement. In cases of severe acidosis where the plasma bicarbonate is less than 15 mEq/1, one may have to administer sodium bicarbonate infusions or oral sodium bicarbonate.

Hyperkalaemia

Treat hyperkalaemia with insulin and dextrose and at the same time start the patient on Resonium A.

Anaemia

If the patient is anaemic with Hb of 7 gm and less, or if he has symptoms due to anaemia he should be transfused with packed red blood cells. However if the patient has been on regular follow-up by a nephrologist, he should be given injections of Erythropoeitin when Hb is less than 10 gm together with iron supplements.

Phosphate Binders

Calcium carbonate and phosphate binders should be used whenever the serum phosphate exceeds 5 mg/dl. Good control of the serum phosphate will cause an increase in serum calcium and also decrease the incidence of metastatic calcification.

Calcium, Vitamin D Supplements

Calcium supplements are usually given early as many patients have low calcium when GFR is less than 30 ml/min. It is given as calcium carbonate or calcium acetate. Calcium supplements are contraindicated in the presence of severe hyperphosphataemia. The use of synthetic vitamin D analogues will depend on the type and degree of renal osteodystrophy. Patients should probably start Rocaltrol or 1-α-di(OH)-D$_3$ as soon as the serum alkaline phosphatase starts to rise. Some prescribe this earlier, two or three times a week instead of daily.

Blood Pressure Control

Judicious control of blood pressure is important as it may retard the progression of chronic renal failure. Beta blockers form the mainstay of treatment together with calcium channel blockers . Though thiazides are no longer of use as diuretics when the GFR is less than 30 ml/min, they are still useful as vasodilators.

For patients with renal failure with serum creatinine less than 500 micro M/L, ACE inhibitor or Angiotensin Receptor Antagonist (ATRA) can be used to reduce intra-glomerular hypertension due to Glomerular Hyperfiltration. Monitor serum potassium and renal function.

Once serum creatinine exceeds 500 micro M/L, ACE inhibitor or ATRA is withdrawn as the danger of hyperkalaemia is increased with worsening renal failure.

Vitamins

Multivitamin and iron supplements are usually prescribed.

Investigations

During investigations, the patient should not be dehydrated. Blood taking in the forearm must be avoided as it may be difficult to create arteriovenous fistulae later if the forearm veins are traumatised or thrombosed.

Sympathy

Remember that the patient is human and you must be too. Show an interest in him. Ask about the food he eats. Enquire about his appetite, his fluid allowance, his sleeping pattern and even his sex life. Listen to his feelings and his fears. Be aware of depression and suicidal tendencies.

Some patients go through a phase of **denial** before they can **accept** their illness. They suffer from **reactive depression** and may require psychiatric counselling.

CHAPTER 26

Dialysis

A patient should be considered for dialysis or transplantation
as soon as it is clear that he or she has chronic renal failure,
usually when serum creatinine is about 500 micro mol/L.
Remember to screen patients for Hepatitis B, C and HIV
infection so that precautions can be taken in positive patients.

Dialysis is usually started when the serum creatinine is about
800 to 900 micro mol/L though occasionally it is indicated
on symptomatic grounds at an earlier stage. The aim should
be to start dialysis before complications of uraemia occur
(pericarditis, nausea and vomiting), so that it should be possible
for a patient to continue full-time employment.

SELECTION

Acceptance policies vary considerably in different countries.
Some countries accept any patient while many others, because
of financial restrictions, select patients based on age, medical,
economic and other factors.

CENTRE DIALYSIS

Centre dialysis in the Singapore General Hospital is usually
required for the initiation of dialysis and for a short period
after transplantation. Home dialysis patients with complications
such as hypertension, vascular access difficulties and severe

infections also need to be dialysed at the Centre. Such complications require a high staff-patient ratio.

HOME DIALYSIS

This is the best option for the patient on dialysis. The patient can dialyse himself after office hours at his own convenience with the aid of his spouse or partner. Employers are happier and such patients are more productive compared to those on centre or self dependency dialysis. In Singapore the set-up for home dialysis which includes the dialysis machine and water treatment unit (reverse osmosis or deioniser) cost about S$30 000 to S$40 000, with a monthly maintenance expenditure for disposables like dialysers, blood-lines and dialysate which together cost about S$1500. It is obvious therefore that not many can afford to dialyse at home.

SELF DEPENDENCY DIALYSIS CENTRES

These centres are developed in most countries to provide a more convenient dialysis location for patients who cannot dialyse at home. To keep costs down, emphasis is placed on self dialysis with a low staff-patient ratio. This policy also retains the advantages of home dialysis in placing the responsibility for care on the patient himself, with a consequent better survival and rehabilitation rate. However, nowadays in Singapore, many patients opt for Assisted Dialysis in the various centres which include those run by the National Kidney Foundation (NKF) or the Kidney Dialysis Foundation (KDF) or the other private dialysis centres where patients are dialysed by the staff in these centres without the need for a spouse or helper, though at a higher cost than the self dependency dialysis centres. Assisted dialysis frees the spouse or family member from turning up at the dialysis centre thrice weekly.

In a few cases, there may be difficulties related to access, or to cramps and hypotension on dialysis but for the majority it provides a reliable and effective form of renal replacement therapy. Haemodialysis is usually performed 3 times per week for 4 hours per session. With newer techniques (high flux dialysis) using special membranes and more sophisticated machines, and with AV fistulae with good blood flow rates, haemodialysis can now be shortened to only $3\frac{1}{2}$ hours. Newer membranes which are more biocompatible have been introduced recently and will doubtless make their impact on the local scene.

Medical Problems still present in Patients on Dialysis

1. **Itch,** sometimes intense and generalised, is often still a problem for the patient on dialysis. A soothing aqueous cream and antihistamines may help. Some patients may respond to a course of ultraviolet therapy.

2. **Bone disease** is still a problem and this is often related to the length of dialysis though most patients will have histological changes on bone biopsy. Some will have radiological changes of osteomalacia or hyperparathyroidism. Patients with renal bone disease will require control of serum calcium and phosphate with calcium carbonate or calcichew. Vitamin D analogues may also be required. Some patients may require partial parathyroidectomy if they do not respond to Vitamin D therapy. These are patients with elevated serum calcium and high serum alkaline phosphatase levels with severe changes of osteodystrophy on skeletal survey. Serum parathyroid levels are also high in these individuals. Nowadays, even in the absence of radiological evidence of renal osteodystrophy, we tend to start our patients on a small dose of 1,25-dihydroxycholecalciferol (Rocaltrol), 0.25 micro gm once

daily on alternate days. Patients with normal liver function can be treated with 1-α-(OH)-D$_3$.

Osteomalacia may not respond to Vitamin D therapy especially in the case of aluminium induced osteomalacia. This is the result of aluminium in tap water and such patients run the risk of developing dialysis dementia. In our unit, since the introduction of reverse osmosis and deionisers to treat our dialysate water, the incidence of dialysis dementia and aluminium induced osteomalacia has become a thing of the past.

3. **Anaemia:** Most patients on regular haemodialysis can tolerate Hb of 8 gm reasonably well. They are transfused if Hb drops below 7 gm or when they have symptoms of anaemia. The advent of human recombinant DNA erythropoeitin has been a boon for patients with anaemia. Most patients are now on it, maintaining Hb level of 10 gm or more. Patients should be on erythropoeitin even before they start dialysis to keep Hb between 10–12 gm. Iron supplements have to be given too.

4. **Hypertension:** In most patients, hypertension is controlled by salt and water depletion by dialysis as well as diet and strict fluid control. About 30% to 40% of patients will still require antihypertensive medication. Control of salt and water related hypertension is important, as patients with left ventricular ejection fraction less than 50% have a high risk of dying from cardiac complication and are not candidates for renal transplant.

5. **Hepatitis:** An effective vaccine has now been developed and those at risk of Hepatitis B (patients, helpers, nurses and doctors) are now routinely immunised. Hepatitis C remains a problem.

6. Apart from the above, patients on dialysis are still prone to **infections** like lung infections and septicaemia.

Septicaemia is often due to contamination during needling of the arteriovenous (AV) fistulae.

7. Finally, as a result of accelerated atherogenesis, arteriosclerosis and hypertension, they are prone to **myocardial infarction** and **cerebrovascular accidents.**

PRINCIPLES INVOLVED IN HAEMODIALYSIS

Dialysis is a process which separates solutes dissolved in water across a semipermeable membrane.

In haemodialysis the patient's blood is let out of his body where it is treated with anticoagulant (heparin) to prevent it from clotting and passed over a semipermeable membrane in the dialyser (artificial kidney) through which exchange of solutes (dialysis) takes place. The exchange occurs across the membrane of the artificial kidney into a solution called the dialysate which has a composition similar to a solution of the body's salts but without any of the waste products.

By means of osmosis and diffusion the waste products of metabolism like urea, creatinine, and potassium which are at a higher concentration in the blood compartment of the artificial kidney pass across the membrane into the dialysate compartment since the latter has a lower concentration of these substances.

During the process of haemodialysis the blood from the patient flows continuously through the dialyser while fresh dialysate is passed through it on the other side of the membrane so that a high gradient of toxic substance is always present on the blood side. The blood returning to the patient after passing through the dialyser is almost devoid of toxic substances accumulated in renal failure.

HAEMOFILTRATION

Excess water from the patient's body is removed by means of haemofiltration using a special dialyzer. A pressure gradient is generated across the membrane using a pump which raises the pressure in the blood compartment, causing more water to be lost through the membrane and into the dialysis compartment.

Hemodiafiltration is a useful procedure for patients with unstable BP and fluid overload as we can remove excess fluid and dialyse the patient as well in spite of the low BP. Hemofiltration and Hemodiafiltration are referred to as continuous renal replacement therapy (CRRT), ideal for patients with Acute Renal Failure in ICU setting.

Vascular Access and How It is Made Possible

In order to get blood out of the patient repeatedly to pass through the artificial kidney machine and back into the body after it has been cleansed, a vascular access is necessary. Put simply, the access is a point of entry into the bloodstream so the patient can be connected to the machine.

The commonest form of access is the arteriovenous (AV) fistula usually done over the wrist. This involves a small operation to join the radial artery with a vein in the arm. The vein would increase in size and develop a thick wall after 3 to 6 weeks. It is then very easy to put a needle into this vein and connect the patient to the machine.

Nowadays for immediate access, an internal jugular catheter is inserted. It is a catheter which is inserted into the internal jugular vein by the side of the neck. This method of access is a temporary measure which provides immediate access for dialysis while the AV fistula which is usually done about the same time matures. The internal jugular catheter cannot be used beyond a few weeks as it tends to get blocked by clotted blood or the site of insertion gets infected. An alternative is the perm-catheter which lasts longer.

Most kidney doctors usually electively have an AV fistula created for the patient when his serum creatinine level is about 500 micro mol/L since it takes about 6 weeks to mature and be ready for needling. This will obviate the need for an internal jugular catheter. The patient is usually started on dialysis when the serum creatinine level is around 1000 micro mol/L depending on whether he has symptoms or other complications of end stage kidney failure by then.

Types of Dialysers (Artificial Kidneys)

1. The hollow fibre dialyser: In this dialyser blood is passed through thousands of minute hollow fibres of membrane around which dialysate (dialysis solution) flows.
2. The flat plate dialyser: Here membranes are stacked together like a sandwich with spaces in between through which dialysate and blood flow in different compartments.

These dialysers though said to be disposable can in fact be reused for 3 to 6 times or more after washing and sterilising at the end of each use.

DIALYSATE

Dialysate is the fluid or solution used for dialysis. For haemodialysis the concentrated dialysate is mixed with 30 to 40 times its volume of water by means of a proportioning pump. The dialysate after mixing is warmed to body temperature and its composition checked by special meters as it passes into the dialysis machine before going into the dialyser.

The Tap Water Used for Haemodialysis

In Singapore, as in most centres, the water used for dialysis has to be treated by reverse osmosis or passed through deionisers to get rid of impurities in the water, especially aluminium. If accumulated in the body of patients with kidney failure, aluminium may cause a degenerative disease of the brain (dialysis dementia) whereby the patient behaves abnormally, has slurred speech, facial distortions, develops repeated convulsions and finally dies. The accumulated aluminium also results in aluminium bone disease which causes bone pain and fractures.

EQUIPMENT REQUIRED FOR HAEMODIALYSIS

The patient will require a haemodialysis machine with a built-in monitoring system and various sets of pumps; the dialyser or artificial kidney; lines for letting out and returning blood to the patient; dialysate or dialysis solution, water treatment unit (deionser or reverse osmosis) and vascular access for the patient (usually an AV fistula).

Functions of the Monitoring System in the Dialysis Machine

The monitoring system ensures a series of automatic checks such that the dialysis procedure is safe for the patient. It incorporates a system of alarms which will go off if a fault is detected.

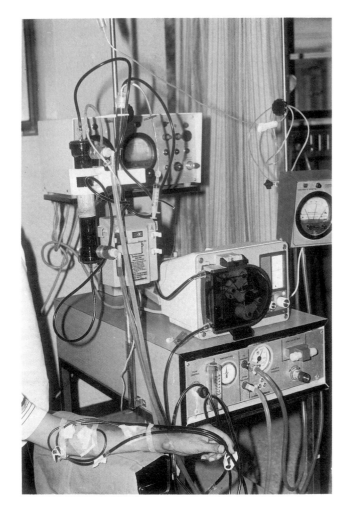

Fig. 26.1   A haemodialysis machine with built-in monitors

The following checks are made by the monitoring system:

1. The dialyser is not leaking blood into the dialysate compartment. This can occur if there is a break in the dialyser membrane. The membranes are very thin (ranging from 5–40 microns depending on the type of membrane used). The diameter of the pores in the membrane ranges

from 1–7 nano metres depending on the type of membrane used.

2. No bubbles are returning to the patient in the venous line as the entry of air into the vein can cause death through air embolism. A bubble trap is usually installed in the system and the presence of air would set off an alarm system.

3. The temperature of the dialysate must be the same as that of the normal body temperature. This is recorded by a temperature gauge.

4. The composition of the dialysate must be correct. This is checked by a conductivity meter.

5. The blood pressure on the arterial and venous lines must be appropriate.

THE EFFECT OF HAEMODIALYSIS ON THE PATIENT

For most patients haemodialysis remains the preferred form of dialysis. It provides a reliable and effective form of kidney replacement therapy. Haemodialysis is usually performed 3 times per week for 4 hours per session.

Initially, most patients will find difficulty with life on haemodialysis. Some may feel unwell and washed out at the end of each dialysis. During dialysis they may have cramps, vomiting or hypotension. These effects are due to the changes occurring in the composition of his body fluids. However, most patients get over these effects after a few weeks. The majority of patients will have the feeling that they have been given a new lease of life. Gone are the symptoms of end stage renal failure, the worse being the nausea and vomiting, not to mention the shortness of breath, giddiness, tiredness and general malaise. Food takes on a new taste and everything in their body seems to be working again.

DIETARY RESTRICTIONS FOR A PATIENT ON HAEMODLALYSIS

The patient still has to observe certain dietary restrictions very strictly.

He is allowed to take normal amounts of meat and carbohydrates but he must restrict potassium, salt and water in his diet. This is because he can still retain lethal amounts of potassium, salt and water in between dialysis. He must avoid all foodstuff containing potassium, some of these being fruits and vegetables. Fruits include preserved fruits such as jams and other preserves. Citrus fruits, especially oranges and grapes are worst. Our local specially, the durian, has claimed many a life on dialysis, as it has particularly high potassium content. Patients who cannot resist its temptation and take a few seeds can meet with sudden death due to arrhythmias induced by severe hyperkalaemia. The only fruits patients can take as a concession are apples and pears, as their potassium content are much lower. However, these too have to be taken sparingly. Phosphate containing foodstuff too have to be reduced.

Vegetables to be taken must be boiled and the water containing the extracted potassium poured away before the vegetable is eaten.

Patients on haemodialysis hardly pass more than about 200 to 300 ml of urine, some even less. Water sometimes accumulates very rapidly in between dialysis. This water is from the food and drinks ingested, as well as the result of the body's metabolic process. In fact, in most patients, accumulation of excess water in the body is due to failure in observing the rules regarding salt and water restriction. Despite being told to reduce their salt intake and restrict the total amount of fluid intake to not more than 500 ml a day, some patients could not help breaking these rules. The recalcitrant ones are those who die suddenly from pulmonary oedema, causing them to drown in their own fluids, which is a terrible way of dying.

Uncontrolled intake of salt and water in a dialysis patient will also cause the patient to develop very high blood pressure which can lead to heart failure, or the bursting of a blood vessel in the brain causing cerebral haemorrhage and death.

Patients in danger of death from fluid overload can have the fluid removed by ultrafiltration through the haemodialysis machine if they go to the hospital in time. This method of fluid removal however will cause severe cramps and unpleasant hypotension especially if more than 2 litres of fluid are removed. The result is that the patient feels terrible but hopefully more compliant the next time.

THE PSYCHOLOGICAL EFFECTS ON THE DIALYSIS PATIENT

For some patients, the thought of being on dialysis for the rest of their lives or until they can get a kidney transplant may mean the end of the world for them and some may even become suicidal. This is especially so in younger patients who find it more difficult to accept a rigid and restricted lifestyle. There is great stress on family members and in some cases, marriages break up and children who are already neglected by a parent's illness prior to the time of dialysis are finally left destitute when the family breaks up.

Many have decreased earnings and others may already have lost their jobs because of their illness. Many too would have to give up whatever social life they previously had as their leisure hours are now occupied by the thrice weekly dialysis.

In those who are dependent on a helper, usually the spouse, he or she is also similarly tied down by the dialysis schedule. Added to all the above problems, males become impotent and females lose their libido, both of which are due to poisonous wastes retained in kidney failure affecting their sexual glands.

Some patients rebel against and refuse to accept the fact that they have kidney failure. Given time however, and support from the medical staff, most finally accept their fate and learn to come to terms with their illness. In fact, these very same patients are the ones who sometimes ironically turn out to be model patients and strict disciplinarians of the various impositions on their new lifestyle.

Most patients therefore do overcome the initial trauma, fears and resentment regarding their illness. They adapt very well and their courage has to be admired. They bear testimony to the belief that the human spirit is indefatigable and indomitable. On a cheerful note, they can also plan to travel abroad as many dialysis units overseas do accommodate visiting patients. For the dialysis patient, it is of utmost importance that he dialyses and maintains himself well in preparation for the day when he should be called up to receive a cadaver transplant..

HALLMARKS OF A WELL DIALYSED PATIENT

The patient who is well dialysed should:
* have a sense of well-being
* have well controlled blood pressure
* absence of heart failure
* haemoglobin of more than 10 gm
* absence of bone disease and neuropathy
* pre-dialysis serum creatinine less than 500 micro mol/L and Kt/V > 1.4

PRINCIPLES OF PERITONEAL DIALYSIS

The peritoneum is a membrane lining the stomach and the intestines. It forms an apron that lies freely in the abdominal cavity. Its rich blood supply allows us to use it for exchange of substances in and out of the body. For the purpose of dialysis, the peritoneal membrane acts as the dialysis membrane. Waste products carried in the blood vessels of the peritoneum would diffuse across the membrane into the dialysate which is infused into the abdominal cavity. Again, by means of principles of osmosis and diffusion, waste products like urea, creatinine and excess potassium which are at a higher concentration in

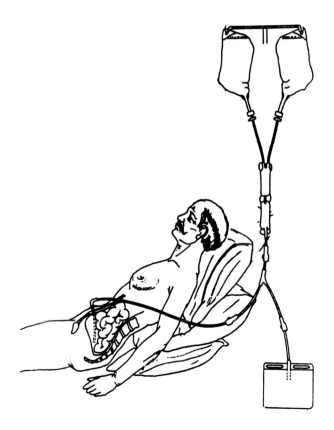

Fig. 26.2 Diagram of a patient on peritoneal dialysis

the blood of patients with renal failure will diffuse into the dialysate in the abdominal cavity and can be drained out.

A flexible catheter called a Tenckhoff Catheter is used for peritoneal dialysis. It is inserted into the peritoneal cavity by means of a sterile technique with aseptic precautions under anaesthetic. The dialysate fluid is then run into the abdomen via the catheter and out again after exchange of waste products has taken place. Each cycle (run-in and run-out of dialysate plus period allowed for diffusion to take place) takes about 1 hour. Usually after 2 to 3 days the patient feels much better with this treatment.

This form of dialysis can be used for the patient who is awaiting the maturation of his AV fistula prior to haemodialysis. It can also be used for the patient with acute renal failure due to septicaemia or drugs where he only requires a few dialyses before kidney function returns. Acute peritoneal dialysis is seldom practised nowadays, most physicians prefer acute hemodialysis or CRRT (Pg 305).

The Tenckhoff Catheter

For the patient who requires long-term peritoneal dialysis (continuous ambulatory peritoneal dialysis or CAPD), a Tenckhoff catheter is used. It is soft and flexible and is made of non-irritating Silastic. It is inserted under anaesthesia in the operating theatre. The correct insertion is important for long-term catheter survival and for avoidance of infection at the site of catheter insertion.

Dialysate used for Patients on Peritoneal Dialysis

The dialysate (dialysis fluid) is sterile and it is supplied in 1- or 2-litre polythene bags. It is a buffered solution of salts like the haemodialysis fluid but is different because of its high glucose content. The glucose is necessary for the removal of fluid from the patient.

The presence of glucose in the dialysate will cause water from the bloodstream to be drawn into the peritoneal cavity by means of osmosis. In this way the patient can get rid of excess fluid which causes swelling of his body.

Continuous Ambulatory Peritoneal Dialysis (CAPD)

There are 2 forms of peritoneal dialysis. Acute peritoneal dialysis is used for intermittent or once-only dialysis. Chronic peritoneal dialysis is employed when the patient requires continuous dialysis and is called CAPD.

In CAPD, the patient performs a slow but continuous exchange using a Tenckhoff catheter, in contrast to acute peritoneal dialysis where hourly exchange is the rule.

CAPD is a form of treatment alternative to haemodialysis for end stage renal failure. The procedure involves exchanging 2 litres of dialysate 4 times a day. This is done daily and at each exchange the bag is rolled up and worn until the next exchange. The patient walks about and does his work until the next exchange when the bag is disconnected and a new one connected and run in.

It has no capital expenditure as the patient does not require a machine and the only disposables are the bags of dialysate. The monthly recurrent expenditure is about S$1,200.

It is simple to use since a patient usually learns the technique within 2 weeks, and the low intrinsic costs have made CAPD popular with many patients. The major disadvantage is the frequent episodes of peritonitis. These can be treated with antibiotics. Control of infection by better exchange techniques and by microbiological filters has reduced the incidence of infection. Lately, the introduction of the ultra bag to check infection in CAPD patients has dramatically reduced the peritonitis rates (1 episode in 44 patient months).

CAPD is a better form of dialysis for patients with kidney failure due to diabetes mellitus. A diabetic on haemodialysis runs the risk of blindness because of the heparin used for haemodialysis which may cause bleeding in his eyes, a tendency arising from diabetic retinopathy. This usually occurs in patients whose kidneys are affected by diabetes.

CAPD is also less strenuous to the heart. It is gentler, unlike hemodialysis where there is an initial run-off of 100 ml of blood into the artificial kidney which may precipitate hypotension in patient with heart disease (commoner among diabetics). Therefore CAPD is recommended for the elderly especially those with ischemic heart disease.

For diabetics on CAPD, there is the additional advantage of administering insulin intra-peritoneally with more physiological absorption compared to subcutaneous route of insulin where there is wider fluctuation of insulin levels.

Automated Peritoneal Dialysis

Apart from CAPD, Chronic Peritoneal Dialysis can also be performed at night when the patient is asleep, using an automated peritoneal dialysis machine. The machine performs the exchanges at night while the patient is asleep. The main advantage is that the patient is free of the burden of dialysing himself in the day time. The expenditure for APD is about $1,600 a month.

SUBSIDY FOR DIALYSIS

The National Policy is to promote the growth of peritoneal dialysis (PD) since this is more cost effective and is an equally viable alternative compared to hemodialysis. As of 1st Dec 2001, both CAPD and APD are subsidized by Government. Patients will have subsidized hemodialysis only if they are found to be unsuitable for PD or medical prounds.

PROGNOSIS FOR PATIENTS ON DIALYSIS

Mortality varies from 5% annually for 20- to 40-year-old patients to 15% annually for those over 60 years. Cause of death is usually due to heart attack, stroke or infection. Only 15% of patients are classified as unfit for full or part-time work on medical grounds. However the typical dialysis patient is anaemic and as a consequence cannot sustain hard physical effort. Hopefully as the cost of human recombinant DNA erythropoeitin becomes more affordable, anaemia of renal failure may be less of a problem and patients with Hb of about 12 gm or more would be able to sustain hard physical effort.

CHAPTER 27

Renal Transplantation

In Singapore, the first cadaver renal transplant was performed in 1970. The first living related donor transplant was performed in 1976.

For cadaver transplants the graft survival rate is 89% for the first year, 85% for the fifth year, and 77% for the tenth year.

For living related donor transplants the graft survival rate is 98% at one year, 92% at 5 years and 82% at 10 years. Table 27.1 shows the number of kidney transplants performed in Singapore.

Our transplant survival rates are comparable to those of advanced centres elsewhere.

Parents and siblings sharing 1 or 2 haplotypes are preferred in living donor transplantation as transplants from relatives with zero matched haplotypes have only the success rate similar to those of cadaver kidneys.

Successful live donation is often gratifying to the donor. Apart from the slight inevitable perioperative risk, the donor suffers no shortening of life or adverse effects on the quality of life. We have had living related renal donors from all walks of life and apart from mild hypertension in a few who are over 50 years which could well be unrelated to renal donation, none of our donors have suffered any adverse effects as a result of their donation.

Table 27.1 Number of kidney transplants performed in Singapore (1970–2001)

| Year | Living Related | Cadaveric | | | Total |
		Local Transplant	Overseas Transplant	Total Cadaveric	
1970	–	1	–	1	1
1971	–	2	–	2	2
1972	–	3	–	3	3
1973	–	2	–	2	2
1974	–	6	–	6	6
1975	–	3	–	3	3
1976	1	3	–	3	4
1977	2	–	–	–	2
1978	10	2	–	2	12
1979	14	–	–	–	14
1980	18	–	–	–	18
1981	15	–	–	–	15
1982	17	8	–	8	25
1983	18	7	18	25	43
1984	12	16	8	24	36
1985	15	1	–	1	16
1986	14	15	5	20	34
1987	12	16	2	18	30
1988	4	23	2	25	29
1989	1	26	2	28	29
1990	11	45	4	49	60
1991	14	36	4	40	54
1992	18	60	17	77	95
1993	24	32	2	34	58
1994	16	84	45	129	145
1995	11	53	26	79	90
1996	12	44	14	58	70
1997	8	25	–	25	33
1998	15	42	14	56	71
1999	13	42	20	62	75
2000	10	54	14	68	78
2001	18	44	10	54	72
TOTAL	323	695	207	902	1225

A patient who is to be transplanted should be mentally and physically prepared. All correctable medical and surgical problems should be attended to while the patient is still on dialysis. This may involve treatment for peptic ulceration or dental clearance as such measures will help to minimise morbidity and mortality.

LIVING RELATED DONOR

Within a family, HLA typing clearly separates siblings into 2, 1 or 0 haplotype matches. This allows the prediction of 95% or 84% 1-year graft survival for 2 or 1 haplotype matches respectively and hence the selection of the best donor. A transplant from a parent to a child has a 84% 1-year graft survival because a child inherits only one haplotype from each of his parents.

CADAVER DONOR

HLA-A and HLA-B matching confers a small but definite benefit. The B locus is probably more important than the A locus. DR locus matching confers an additional benefit.

A prerequisite for a successful graft is ABO compatibility, and a negative cross-match of donor T lymphocytes and recipient sera using a sensitive direct cytotoxic technique. Kidneys are harvested from brain dead donors. It is important to maintain the blood pressure of the potential donor to ensure adequate urine flow (about 60 ml/hour) as this will increase the likelihood of a viable donor kidney. When a cadaver kidney has been obtained it is cooled by simple perfusion with a hyper-osmolar solution and then left at 4°C prior to transplantation. Over 25% of grafts run a course of acute tubular necrosis for 1 to 2 weeks.

TISSUE TYPING

In our body is a particular series of closely linked genes called the Major Histocompatibility Complex (MHC). In humans, the MHC codes for proteins or antigens called the Human Leukocyte Antigen (HLA) that are important in kidney transplant matching. There are two principal classes of HLA. The class I HLA genes are named HLA-A, HLA-B and HLA-C, and the class II HLA genes are named HLA-DR, -DQ and -DP. Each HLA gene has multiple alternate forms called alleles. Each person inherits one allele of each HLA gene from his father and one allele of each HLA gene from his mother. Thus, each of us will have two sets of HLA gene alleles, i.e. two HLA-A alleles, two HLA-B alleles, two HLA-C alleles, two HLA-DR alleles, etc. Because each gene has many alleles, this leads to an extremely large number of possible combinations, making it difficult to have matching HLA types for unrelated individuals.

PATTERN OF INHERITANCE OF HLA TYPES

Because HLA genes are closely linked, they are inherited as a set of HLA-A, -B, -C, -DR, and -DQ alleles, called a haplotype. Each child will inherit one haplotype from the father and one from the mother. A child will therefore share one haplotype or at least 50% of HLA with each of his parents. Between siblings, they have a one in four chance of identical HLA (inherit the same haplotypes from both parents), a one in two chance of sharing half the HLA (inherit the same haplotype from one parent), and a one in four chance of completely non-identical HLA (inherit different haplotypes from both parents). Apart from parents and siblings, HLA typing matches are less common because of the diversity of HLA gene alleles. In practice, there should be at least a 25% match before living related donor transplant can be done, which would include the parents and some of the siblings (Fig. 27.1).

(Above two sections by courtesy of Diana Teo)

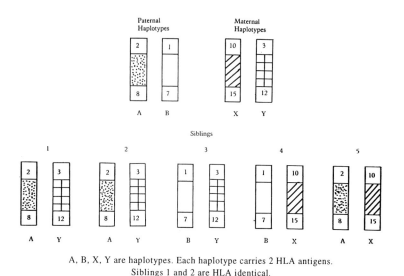

A, B, X, Y are haplotypes. Each haplotype carries 2 HLA antigens.
Siblings 1 and 2 are HLA identical.

Fig. 27.1   Human Leukocyte Antigen (HLA) segregation within a family

ABO BLOOD GROUPING IN KIDNEY TRANSPLANT

All of us have a certain type of blood group on our red blood cells. For a kidney transplant to be successful the blood group between the donor and the recipient must be compatible, otherwise the transplanted kidney will be rejected very quickly by the recipient's body. Blood grouping rules apply to both cadaver and living related transplants.

The various blood groups are A, B, O, and AB. O is the universal donor and can give to O, A, B, AB but can only receive from O.

AB is the universal acceptor. It can accept from O, A, B, AB but can only give to AB.

A can receive from O or A and can give to A and AB. B can receive from O or B and can give to B and AB.

All this means that if the patient has O group he can only receive a kidney from an O donor. If he is A, he can receive from O and A. If he is B, he can receive from O and B. If he is AB he can receive from O, A, B and AB.

THE MIXED LYMPHOCYTE REACTION

This is a test to determine whether the recipient's lymphocytes will react very strongly to those of the donor's. If there is a very strong reaction, it may not be wise to do the transplant as there is a high possibility that the transplanted kidney will be rejected.

In this test, the prospective donor and the recipient's lymphocytes are mixed together and incubated. The strength of the recipient's reaction to the prospective donor is measured. A strong mixed lymphocyte reaction suggests that the donor's cells are not compatible with the recipient's and there is a good chance of the kidney being rejected.

FITNESS TO DONATE A KIDNEY

The kidney donor for living related transplantation must be at least 21 years old so that he can give his consent for kidney donation. He should not be more than 60 years old as old people tend to have very stiff and thick wall arteries (atherosclerosis). In kidney transplant the blood vessels of the donor's kidney has to be stitched to those of the recipient. If the blood vessels are atherosclerotic it makes the surgeon's job very difficult and dangerous as the vessels are more likely to tear during the operation. In addition, older people tend to have hypertension and kidneys that may be already slightly damaged by the process of ageing.

The donor must be healthy and have no illness or systemic disease like diabetes and hypertension that might already have caused damage to their kidneys. They must of course not have kidney disease themselves.

Is it safe for a parent or sibling to donate a kidney? Will it do any harm? What about people who do heavy work? Can young women marry and have children after giving away one kidney?

These are the questions that are often asked at the same time by several anxious relatives of the patient with kidney failure. A normal person has two kidneys but one kidney is sufficient to enable one to lead a normal life. The other kidney acts like a reserve. It is like a car with 4 spare tyres. If the 4 spare tyres are removed the car can still function normally. Or expressed another way, one can say that the two kidneys represent 200% kidney function. So, after donating a kidney the donor can still lead a normal life with no restriction whatsoever. He can continue to do heavy work. In the case of a woman she can still marry and have babies. However, should the donor meet with an accident and the remaining kidney is damaged he runs the risk of kidney failure, since his other kidney which acts as a reserve has been donated earlier.

Complications of Live Kidney Donation

Apart from the slight unavoidable risk which occurs in any major operation, the donor suffers no shortening of life or adverse effects on the quality of life. We have had living related renal donors from all walks of life and apart from mild hypertension in a few donors who were over 50 years which could well be unrelated to renal donation none of the donors have suffered any adverse effects as a result of their donation.

The donor would experience some pain over the operative wound which can be relieved by injections of pethidine. He has to stay in hospital for about a week and after that would be given medical leave to rest at home. He should be back at work within a month's time. Once a year he has to go for a renal check-up where the blood pressure, urine and blood are checked to make sure that the remaining kidney is well.

Social Pressure on a Relative to Donate Kidney

In Singapore, as we are short of cadaver donors and dialysis is expensive, the patient's relatives (parents, brothers and sisters) have to be approached by the doctors regarding volunteers for living related kidney donation in order to save the life of the patient. A lot of social pressure may be brought to bear upon the potential kidney donor, sometimes conflicting pressures.

A brother or sister may want to donate a kidney to another brother or sister but may face parental objection, especially if the parents tend to be elderly. On the other hand, a brother or sister may be pressurised to donate by the parents. Married people may face objections from in-laws. A sister may want to donate to a brother but her mother-in-law may object. Similarly a wife or husband may object to a spouse donating a kidney to a sibling. Even boy friends, girl friends and fiancees/fiances have been known to object.

In general married people face more social pressure in giving a kidney, particularly when they have dependent children. There is always the fear on the spouse's part that if something should happen to the donor the family may be left without a father (sole bread winner) or mother (home-maker). Family conflicts can result in marriages breaking up. Sometimes between parents and children, loyalties may be divided to provide for a single child who is sick while depriving the other offspring at home of a parent. Also parents would have to face up to the possibility that despite their sacrifice the kidney may not function usefully and all will have been in vain.

Finally, there may be conflict between siblings or even between parents as to who should give a kidney. Some may argue about the effect of donation on a career or the future of child bearing on an unmarried potential donor.

The stand of kidney doctors with regard to living related donor transplantation and what they tell potential donors

Kidney doctors always stress to the family that renal donation is voluntary and there should be no pressure on a particular individual to donate his or her kidney. Any social pressure from relatives on the potential donor is strongly discouraged. Potential donors are informed of the various tests they must pass in order to be considered suitable donors. The doctors cannot guarantee that the transplant will always be successful. There will be a few transplanted kidneys that will not work. Donors would be told about transplant survival rate. It would also be explained to them that donating a kidney would mean loss of renal reserve.

Successful live donation would of course be gratifying to the donor. He or she would have given a new lease of life to a loved one. Apart from slight perioperative risks the donor should suffer no shortening of life or adverse effects on the quality of life.

Spouse to Spouse Renal Transplant

During the last few years we have implemented the Spouse to Spouse Transplant Programme. This is the only form of living unrelated transplant allowed in Singapore. It is heartening and justifiable as married couples share an emotional bond though they are not blood relatives. With the advent of Cyclosporine A and the improved success rates of cadaver transplant on CyA, as long as there is ABO blood group compatibility, spouse to spouse transplant is justifiable and can be performed. We have so far done about 33 patients with 100% success rates.

Assessment of Donor for Living Related Transplantation

The potential donor has to undergo a very thorough and vigorous investigation to make sure that both his kidneys are healthy. If there is the slightest doubt, his kidney will not be taken from him. He must be in good health and have no history of kidney disease, hypertension, diabetes mellitus, cancer or any other disease. He will be assessed psychologically and mentally to ensure that he fully comprehends the nature of the donation, that there are no social pressures on him to donate and that he is donating voluntarily out of love and consideration for the patient. He will undergo a thorough physical examination. The urine and blood tests performed on him must be normal. There must be no protein or blood in the urine. He must have no evidence of renal disease and have normal creatinine clearance.

The ABO blood group between the donor and the recipient must be compatible. The HLA tissue typing should have at least a 25% match. In addition a cross match is performed between the white blood cells (lymphocytes) of the donor and the serum of the recipient. If there are antibodies present in the recipient's serum against the donor's white cells the white cells would be killed by the antibodies. This means that the same antibodies would attack the transplant kidney if it were transplanted in the recipient. Therefore it would not be safe or wise for the donor to donate his kidney which is bound to be rejected by the recipient. All further transplant work-up tests for the particular donor would be discontinued once he is found unsuitable. Another volunteer or the next best volunteer based on the degree of matching of the tissue typing would have to come up for tests.

If the above tests are satisfactory the prospective donor then undergoes an arteriogram to visualise the blood vessels of his kidneys and also to look for any abnormality in the kidneys and to make a decision as to which kidney to remove for the transplant. If all the tests are satisfactory the donor is considered suitable for kidney donation and a date for the transplant operation will be scheduled.

Potential Cadaver Kidney Donors

Donors should not be patients suffering from cancer as cancer may have invaded the kidney and it could be carried over to the recipient with the kidney. The donor should not have infection too as it can be transmitted to the recipient. The cadaver donor should also not be more than 60 years of age. Most donors were patients who had sustained head injuries from road traffic or other accidents. Sometimes bleeding in the brain from various causes can also cause brain death, qualifying the person as a suitable cadaver donor.

The potential donor is therefore someone who has had an accident or damage to the brain with no possibility of recovery and is being maintained on a respirator to ventilate the lungs. It is important that the potential donor be placed on a respirator as it pumps oxygen into the donor's lungs and keeps the heart beating so that blood would flow to the kidneys to keep them functioning, though the donor's brain is already dead (brain dead).

Brain Death

When a person dies it means his brain has ceased to function. The medical term for this is brain death. The beating of the heart and respiration can be taken over by machines but it does not mean that the dead person is still alive. If the machines are turned off the heart and respiration will stop because the dead brain is incapable of supporting these functions.

By testing certain functions of the brain and noting their absence, doctors can pronounce that a person is dead. The criteria for brain death are:

- absence of spontaneous respiration
- fixed and dilated pupils
- no response to pain
- absence of corneal reflex
- absence of gag reflex
- absent doll's eye movement
- no response to the cold caloric test

When all the above criteria are fulfilled the patient can be pronounced brain dead. It means that the brain has been so severely damaged that it is not capable of sustaining life and there is no possibility of its recovery.

Note that the heart can still be beating in a person who is brain dead because the heart muscles can continue to beat for some time after brain death. For the purpose of kidney transplant it is important that the cadaver donor's heart is still beating as it means that blood is still circulating into the kidneys to keep them functioning and producing urine. If the heart has stopped beating for more than an hour, the kidneys which have been deprived of blood during this time would be irreparably damaged and of no use at all in kidney transplantation. This explains why kidneys for transplantation must be removed during the time the person is brain dead rather than wait till the time when the heart stops beating because they will be useless by then.

Kidney Transplant Legislation

In most countries most of the transplanted kidneys are from cadaver donors but in Asian countries most of our transplanted kidneys come from living-related donors. There is sadly a lack of cadaver donors because relatives have not been willing to give consent for kidney donation for various cultural and other reasons. These kidneys which are buried or cremated actually go to waste because they could be used to save many Singaporeans who die needlessly because they are unable to get cadaver kidney transplants. It is a tragedy as the majority are young, aged between 30 and 40. Many are married and are fathers or mothers of very young children. Many are also sole bread winners at the peak of their lives. The majority die due to a lack of cadaver kidneys.

The Medical Therapy, Education & Research Act (MTA) was passed in Parliament in 1972 to enable individuals to will their kidneys for transplantation in the event of death. This is called the Opting-in-law. But even though 28,401 individuals had pledged their kidneys, not a single kidney had become available for transplantation. The average number of kidney transplants averaged only about 5 a year.

The government studied this problem and came out with a solution. In 1986, 128 people died from road traffic accidents. To save 100 patients with kidney failure only 50 brain dead cadavers are required because each cadaver has 2 kidneys and a patient with kidney failure needs only one kidney to survive. A law called the Human Organ Transplant Act (Opting-out-law) or HOTA was passed on 16th July 1987 and implemented in January 1988. The Act allows for the removal of kidneys from Singaporeans and Permanent Residents who die from accidents for the purpose of transplant to kidney failure patients, unless they have specifically objected to this in their lifetime. In some countries like France, Austria, Israel and Belgium where this Act is practised, many patients who suffer from kidney failure have been saved. Since the implementation of HOTA, together with the MTA, the number of cadaveric renal transplants has increased. (see Table 27.1)

Preparation of the Patient for Renal Transplant

Usually the patient who is to receive a transplant will be on regular dialysis having been registered among a long list of patients awaiting renal transplants. When there is a potential cadaver donor available, the donor's tissue typing will be performed and the two patients with the closest match with compatible ABO blood group will be called up urgently and prepared for the transplant. One cadaver has two kidneys which means that 2 patients can be transplanted at the same time. The patients are checked to ensure that they have been well dialysed and then prepared for the operation. In addition they are given injections of prednisolone and azathioprine. Cyclosporin A is not given preoperatively for cadaver transplants. It is started only after the transplant operation when the graft starts producing urine. In this way the nephrotoxic effects on the ischaemic graft which is still recovering from acute tubular necrosis is minimised.

The Transplant Operation

During the transplant operation, the cadaver kidney which has been earlier harvested and kept on ice is put into the pelvis of the patient with kidney failure (recipient), low down and to one side of the bladder. The blood vessels of the kidney are joined to the internal iliac artery and the common iliac vein of the recipient. The ureter of the donated kidney is then sewn onto the recipient's urinary bladder. The operation itself takes about one and a half to two hours (Fig. 27.2).

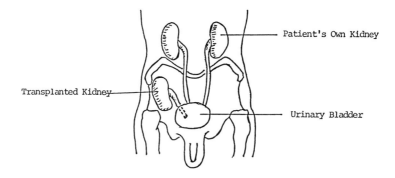

Fig. 27.2   Position of the transplanted kidney

What Happens to the Patient (Recipient) After the Operation?

After the operation the patient is under intensive care. All the urine collected is measured and carefully charted to keep a record of his progress. Usually cadaver transplants take a few days before they can make urine, sometimes up to two weeks. A few may not work at all. During this period the blood urea, creatinine and serum electrolytes are measured everyday. If there is poor urine production by the transplanted kidney the blood tests will still be abnormal and the patient will still continue to require dialysis 3 times a week until the kidney can put out a good amount of urine.

The patient will also receive daily anti-rejection medicine to prevent his body from rejecting the transplant. These drugs are prednisolone, azathioprine and cyclosporin A. If the blood pressure is high he will have to continue taking blood pressure medicine to lower it.

A renal scan is performed the day after the transplant to check that the blood flow through the kidney is adequate and the kidney is well perfused with blood. If there is no blood flow to the kidney the transplant surgeons will have to explore the kidney. Usually the cause is due to a blood clot blocking the blood vessel of the kidney. After removing the clot the kidney will function again.

Even when the kidney is functioning, blood tests have to be performed to watch out for acute rejection which is usually diagnosed by a raised serum creatinine. A renal biopsy of the transplanted kidney may be performed to confirm a diagnosis of acute rejection. If rejection is diagnosed, the patient is given a 3-day course of methylprednisolone. This will usually reverse the rejection process.

Sometimes there may be problems like obstruction of the transplanted kidney or there may be leakage of urine from the ureter of the transplant kidney. An ultrasound examination of the transplanted kidney would have to be performed to determine the cause and site of the obstruction or urinary leakage and if necessary, the transplant surgeon will be called in to explore the kidney with a view to repairing the urine leak or remove the cause of obstruction.

The Donor Nephrectomy on a Live Donor

The kidney is removed from a live donor by means of an operation. The incision is made in the flank to expose the kidney. The blood vessels of the kidney are tied and cut. The kidney is then lifted out of the incision wound, flushed with cold solution and carried to the adjacent operation theatre where the recipient is waiting and then inserted into the recipient's body as for cadaver transplant described before.

The donor's operative wound is sutured and he returns to the ward. The donor should be out of bed after a couple of days and home within 2 weeks.

Immunosuppressive Drugs

During the transplant operation and after, for as long as the transplanted patient is alive, he will have to take his transplant medication faithfully in order to prevent the kidney from being rejected. The medication consists of prednisolone, azathioprine and cyclosporin A. These drugs may predispose the patient to infection. The common sites of infection are in the urine, lungs, skin or bloodstream. The other problem is that there is a definite increase in the tendency to develop cancer in the long term; this risk however is very small.

The other side effects relate to prednisolone, but nowadays, with a tendency to the use of much smaller doses of prednisolone these effects are much decreased. Patients who are on prednisolone develop an increase in the size of their cheeks (moon face). Their appetite increases and they gain weight and become obese. They may also develop high blood pressure, diabetes mellitus, ulcers in the stomach and a condition called avascular necrosis which causes pain in the hip bone. The pain can be relieved by pain relievers but if it gets worse then an operation can be performed to replace the hip with a metal one.

Cyclosporin A is the most important drug used in preventing transplant rejection and though expensive it is being used in countries all over the world because of the tremendous boost it confers on long-term kidney transplant survival. Among some of its disadvantages, apart from prohibitive cost, are its toxicity to the kidney when too high a dose is given and risk of cancer developing in long-term users. Hence it is important to measure the levels of cyclosporin A in the bloodstream so that the dose could be adjusted if the levels are too high in order to try to avoid the toxic effect of the drug. Other side effects of cyclosporin A are increased hair growth (hirsutism), swollen gums, tremors, inflammation of the liver (hepatitis), but the worst as mentioned earlier is nephrotoxicity or toxicity to the kidneys which can cause kidney damage. Hepatitis positive transplant patients should not be put on azathioprine as it is more hepatotoxic than cyclosporin A. They are only on dual therapy with cyclosporine A and prednisolone compared to all the other patients who are on triple therapy consisting cyclosporine A (8 mg/ kg BW), azathioprine (1 mg/kg BW) and prednisolone (20–30 mg) daily.

Tacrolimus (FK 506) (0.25 mg/kg BW), Mycophenolate Mofetil (MMF) (1gm BD) and Rapamycin (2 mg OM) are the newer immunosuppressive agents which are being introduced. Rapamycin can also be used to treat refractory acute rejection. It may limit the development and progression of chronic rejection. (Ref: R N Saunders et al. *Kidney Int.* 2001, **59**: 3–16).

COMPLICATIONS OF KIDNEY TRANSPLANTATION

Early complications are acute rejection, urinary leaks, infections, stomach ulcers and wound infection. Late complications include chronic rejection, avascular necrosis of bone, transplant renal artery stenosis, cancer, infections and recurrent or de novo glomerulonephritis in the transplanted kidney which in some cases can again lead to kidney failure.

Transplant Rejection

Despite the routine use of cyclosporine A, azathioprine and steroids, the careful selection of donors and recipients and the fulfilment of all the prerequisites for successful grafting, rejection occurs and is the major cause of graft failure. In the first 6 months about 20% of cadaver kidneys are rejected as are 10% of related donor kidneys.

Acute rejection is usually diagnosed by a raised serum creatinine without other obvious cause such as obstruction, sepsis, or uncontrolled hypertension due to renal artery stenosis. Sometimes rejection is accompanied by a swollen graft with tenderness, fever and oliguria. A closed biopsy of the graft readily confirms the diagnosis of rejection.

A renogram is useful in assessing renal perfusion of the graft and is useful in diagnosing renal artery thrombosis as a cause of non-function. Ultrasound of the graft too is useful in excluding obstruction due to hydronephrosis causing renal deterioration.

The usual treatment of acute rejection is to give 0.5 gm I.V. boluses of methylprednisolone for 3 days. Antithymocyte or antilymphocyte globulin or OKT3 (monoclonal antibody) is used for severe acute rejection. These are expensive but nonetheless useful in severe acute rejection. Plasmapheresis, graft irradiation, and thoracic duct drainage have been used by other centres but none of these have gained an established place.

Chronic rejection occurs from about 3 to 6 months after transplant. It causes a slow deterioration of graft function and progresses often relentlessly to end stage graft failure over months to years. It is usually associated with proteinuria and hypertension. On biopsy the lesions are usually vascular as opposed to the cellular lesions in acute rejection. There is no treatment for chronic rejection.

Nowadays most centres are using a low dose steroid regimen, ie. 30 mg/day prednisolone initially and reducing to 10 mg/day by the end of 3 months. This is in contrast to the old regimen that starts at 60 mg/day of prednisolone, reducing to 30 mg at 3 months post-graft, and to 10 mg/day at 6 months. Patients on low dose steroids have less morbidity and less avascular necrosis and the long-term graft survival is just as good.

Monoclonal anti-T cell antibody: The use of monoclonal antibody to T cell subsets has been reported to assist the early diagnosis and prediction of rejection. They have also been used to treat acute rejection. But their usefulness may be limited by antibody formation to the monoclonal antibody apart from cost and availability. It should be reserved for patients with severe acute rejection which has not responded to pulse therapy with methylprednisolone.

Anti-Thymocyte Globulin (ATG) is another useful agent for treatment of severe acute rejection.

ADVANTAGES OF TRANSPLANTATION

The quality of life is much better for the patient who has been transplanted as opposed to one on regular haemodialysis. There is greater mobility as he is no longer tied to a kidney machine three times a week. The spouse or partner assisting him on dialysis is also freed of the burden of dialysis. Dialysis only rids the patients of waste products of protein metabolism but it does nothing in terms of the hormonal role of the kidney like producing 1,25-dihydroxycholecalciferol, erythropoietin, and prostaglandins which the transplanted kidney would be capable of doing. The family and working life of the patient is also less disrupted with a transplant compared to the long hours spent on haemodialysis. The patient is also freed from paying for the machine as well as the monthly maintenance.

The only medication required by the patient are prednisolone, azathioprine and cyclosporin A. It is imperative that he remembers to take his medication faithfully, as the omission can cause a prompt rejection of the grafted kidney. Some patients after transplantation may also have to continue taking medication for the control of hypertension. Surely these are minor inconveniences for someone who has been given a new lease of life. An additional bonus is that most men will regain their potency after successful transplantation and women will become fertile and can bear children.

ATRA Therapy in IgA Nephritis

Since ACE inhibitors decrease ACE activity, ACE inhibitor therapy in patients with IgA nephritis would be expected to reduce renal injury in these patients. We have shown that ACEI therapy does lead to decreased proteinuria and retardation of the progression of renal failure in IgA nephritis. In our study we also showed that Angiotension II Receptor Antagonist (ATRA) is as effective as ACEI in decreasing proteinuria and preservation of renal function.[1]

It has been postulated that ACEI/ATRA (ACE inhibitor/ Angiotensin receptor antagonist) may decrease proteinuria in patients with glomerulonephritis by its action on the Glomerular Basement Membrane. We performed a study to examine the relationship between the response of patients with IgA Nephritis (IgA Nx) to ACEI (Enalapril)/ATRA (Losartan) therapy by decreasing proteinuria and its effect on the Selectivity Index (SI) in these patients. Forty one patients with biopsy proven IgA Nx entered a control trial with 21 in the treatment group and 20 in the control group. The entry criteria included proteinuria of 1 gm or more and or renal impairment. Patients in the treatment group received ACEI (5 mg)/ATRA (50 mg) or both with 3 monthly increase in dosage. In the control group, hypertension was treated with atenolol, hydrallazine or methyldopa. After a mean duration of therapy of 13 ± 5 months, in the treatment group there was no significant change in serum creatinine, proteinuria or SI but in the control group, serum creatinine deteriorated from 1.8 ± 0.8 to 2.3 ± 1.1 mg/dl ($p < 0.05$). Among the 21 patients in the treatment group, 10 responded to ACEI/ATRA therapy determined as decrease in proteinuria by 30% (responders) and the other 11 did not (non responders). Among the responders, SI improved from a mean of 0.26 ± 0.07 to 0.18 ± 0.07 ($p < 0.001$) indicating a tendency towards selective proteinuria. This was associated with improvement in serum creatinine from mean 1.7 ± 0.6 to 1.5 ± 0.6 mg/dl ($p < 0.02$) and decrease in proteinuria from mean of 2.3 ± 1.1 g/day to 0.7 ± 0.5 g/day ($p < 0.001$).

After treatment, proteinuria in the treatment group (1.8 ± 1.6 g/day) was significantly less than in the control group (2.9 ± 1.8 g/day) ($p < 0.05$). The post treatment SI in the responder group (0.18 ± 0.07) was better than that of the non responder group (0.33 ± 0.11) ($p < 0.002$). Eight out of 21 patients in the treatment group who had documented renal impairment had improvement in their renal function compared to 2 in the control group ($x^2 = 4.4$, $p < 0.05$). Of the 8 patients in the treatment group who improved their renal function, 3 normalized their renal function.

Our study showed that ACEI/ATRA therapy may be beneficial in patients with IgA Nephritis with renal impairment and non selective proteinuria as such patients may respond to therapy with improvement in protein selectivity, decrease in proteinuria and improvement in renal function. ACEI/ATRA therapy probably modifies pore size distribution by reducing the radius of large nonselective pores, causing the shunt pathway to become less pronounced resulting in less leakage of protein into the urine.

Individual antiproteinuric response to ACEI/ATRA therapy varies depending on ACE gene polymorphism as those with the DD genotype respond better to the antiproteinuric effect of ACEI/ATRA therapy.[2,3] Yoshida[3] in a study examining the role of the deletion polymorphism of the ACE gene in the progression and therapeutic responsiveness of IgA nephropathy using the ACEI lisinopril reported that the ACEI lisinopril significantly decreased proteinuria in the DD genotype patients but not in the II or ID genotype. Similar findings have also been reported by Moriyama.[4]

REFERENCE

1. Woo KT, Lau YK, Wong KS, Chiang GSC. ACE/ATRA therapy decreases proteinuria by improving glomerular permselectivity in IgA nephritis. *Kidney Int.* 2000, **58**:2485–2491.

2. Vleming LJ, van Kooten C, van Dijik M. The D-allele of the ACE gene polymorphism predicts a stronger antiproteinuric response to ACE inhibitors. *Nephrology.* 1998, **4**:143–149.

3. Yoshida H, Mitarai T, Kawamura T. Role of the deletion polymorphism of the angiotensin converting enzyme gene in the progression and therapeutic responsiveness of IgA nephropathy. *J Clin Invest.* 1995, **96**:2162–2169.

4. Moriyama T, Kitamura H, Ochi S. Association of angiotensin I-converting enzyme gene polymorphism with susceptibility to antiproteinuric effect of angiotensin I-converting enzyme inhibitors in patients with proteinuria. *J Am Soc Nephrol.* 1995, **6**:1674–1678.

Index